Diet is a Four Letter Word

About the Author

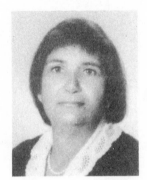

Cole-Webber

Mary Wright lives in Houston, Texas, and runs a large 'flea market' in the center of town. She has two married children, daughter, Bebe, and son, John.

She was brought up in America's Southwest and her fondest childhood memories are of huge, loving family parties with buttered corn, fried chicken and chocolate cake. And the confusing double message that ran along it all, that fat was not a good thing to be. 'Eat up,' she was told on the one hand. 'But don't get fat.'

No wonder it took the author half a lifetime to come to terms with her own self-image, and find a slimming way of indulging her love of good food.

Diet is a
Four Letter Word

Mary Wright's
success with the Duke Diet and
Fitness Program

In association with
Pamela Westland

Eric Bruton Associates Ltd,
Colchester, Essex

First Published 1987

Book design and illustrations by
Slade-Baker & Strange Creative Partnership

British Library Cataloguing in Publication Data

Wright, Mary
    Diet is a four letter word :
    Mary Wright's success with the Duke
    diet and fitness programme.
    1. Reducing diets   2. Physical fitness
    3. Reducing exercises
    I. Title   II. Westland, Pamela
    613.2'5   RM222.2

    ISBN 0-7198-0024-2

Text input by Eric Bruton Associates Ltd.
Typeset by Budget Typesetting Ltd,
Beckenham, Kent.
Printed and bound in Great Britain by
Anchor Brendon Ltd, Tiptree, Colchester,
Essex.

Contents

DEDICATION

To my daughter Bebe, for all her support
when I needed it most. To my son John,who
has my highest admiration and respect. To my
mother Mary and my sister Joanna, whom I
love and cherish. To Pamela, without whose
dedication and hard work this book would
not have come into being, and to David Men-
dell, without whom none of this would have
been possible. And to all of you out there who
are fighting the good fight. You have my
support.

Learning

After a while you learn the subtle
difference between holding a
hand and chaining a soul,

And you learn that love doesn't
mean leaning and company
doesn't mean security.

And you begin to learn that kisses
aren't contracts and presents
aren't promises,

And you begin to accept your defeats
with your head up and your
eyes open, with the grace of an
adult, not the grief of a child,

And you learn to build all your
roads on today because tomorrow's
ground is too uncertain for plans.

After a while you learn that even
sunshine burns if you get too much.

So plant your own garden and decorate
your own soul, instead of waiting
for someone to bring you flowers.

And you learn that you really can endure ....
that you really are strong.

And you really do have worth.

Anon

Introduction

Six years ago I weighed 235 pounds (close to seventeen stones). Now, for a six-foot-two linebacker that's just about right. But for a five-foot-two female person that's very wrong!

Today, I've lost almost ninety pounds and hope to reach my goal of a one hundred pound loss. But if I don't, that will be okay too. You see, I've learned a great deal about myself in those six years, as well as a great deal about dieting. As a matter of fact, when I discovered the Duke Diet and Fitness Center I quit dieting and started learning how to *live* in order to lose weight and keep it off. Because of the knowledge I acquired there about nutrition, behavior, the medical aspects of obesity and the role that fitness must play in my life, I developed a plan for my life which has enabled me to actually reach my goal of weight loss, keep it off, and feel really good about myself.

I am one of those people who has been fat since childhood. I like to say I never weighed under one hundred pounds even when I was born, but am prepared to admit that can't be true. However, what is a fact is that in my mind I have always been fat.

Before I discovered Duke, I had tried just about every diet you can name, including shots of the urine of pregnant women. You remember that one? Of course, along with the shots we were put on a 500-calorie diet and told that these shots would keep us from being hungry. What a laugh that was. I even fasted in the hospital under a doctor's supervision. The only thing I learned from that was that there are more food advertisements on television than all other products put together!

The problem with all of these attempts was that I thought I could 'go on a diet' and when I had lost weight, I 'went off the diet'. I had just never faced the reality which they taught me at Duke: This is your life, and in order to lose weight and maintain the loss you must have a realistic plan for daily living. No more going on and then going off a diet. Duke taught me how to live and enjoy life while maintaining my weight loss.

You know how it is when you have lost weight and people begin to notice you look thinner. The first question they ask is, 'How did you do it?' What they want to hear is, 'Well, I took this magic pill and woke up

9

one morning thin and beautiful.' Sorry folks, there is no magic pill. But there is this book which I have written for all of you out there who need help as I did. I am passing on the message which Duke gave to me and gives to all who come to Durham. This is for those who can't get to the program in person. The people at the Diet and Fitness Center care about you even though you have never met. I and they know what you suffer and we want to help you achieve your goals of weight loss and maintenance. I hope that, for you, this book will be *your* magic pill. It will certainly be the last diet book you will ever have to buy.

Background to the Duke Diet

The Duke Diet which gave me the key to solving my weight problem, and could do the same for you, was originally devised to combat obesity. It has been developed from a research project started in 1969 and headed by Dr Siegried Heyden, the eminent physician and professor at Duke University Medical School in Durham, North Carolina, where he was given free rein for his studies. This diet now has relevance and can be of real benefit to everyone, everywhere who is an overweight person - which is talking about 40 per cent of the population of the United States of America, for a start.

The target Dr Heyden set himself was to construct a diet that would most effectively reduce weight and maintain the health and activity level of patients, whilst keeping within the National/International Standards of 60 grams of protein per day.

As it happens, this was almost exactly the protein level on which Dr Heyden survived healthily as a growing youngster in his native Germany. By what he calls a 'chance observation' Dr Heyden realized that the diet provided by the Air Lift instituted by the three Allied occupying forces during the Berlin Blockade (the United States, the United Kingdom and France), was well under 1000 calories a day and comprised approximately 60 grams of protein. Whilst those people with a garden could supplement the rations with fresh fruit and vegetables, the majority of the population remained healthy on the basic allowance, whilst maintaining their level of activity.

Dr Heyden's recollection of his own feeling of well-being at the time gave him a clue, and led him to the conclusion that this level of nutrition would be a good starting point for his research project.

The project began in a modest way. His first patient was a very obese man whose wife was so concerned about his health (he frequently stopped breathing when he snored at night) that it was ruining her own. Dr Heyden agreed to take up the challenge. By the end of the first week he had four patients. Word of his work got around and within a month or two he had as many as he could handle.

These early patients were all male, mostly maintenance personnel employed at Duke and, it has to be said, all grossly overweight; some weighed as much as 360 pounds (25 stone 10 lb). 'After a few months,' Dr Heyden told me, 'I could predict to a newcomer that using this diet, with the two days of fasting, he could lose up to 60 pounds (4 stone 4 lb) in two months.'

Such astounding results did not escape the notice of the nursing staff at Duke Hospitals. They saw how well the maintenance men were doing, went to Dr Heyden and asked to be included in the program.

What had been unofficially named 'The Working Man's Diet' now had a feminine strand. The Working Woman's Diet was duly launched.

At first the experimental diet was set at 700 calories a day for five days a week, with Saturdays and Sundays designated as fast days. On those two days patients were restricted to non-calorie liquids - water, tea, coffee and calorie-free soft drinks. A tough regime!

In fact, a high liquid intake has always been one of the main tenets of the diet. 'Most people, if they don't eat, don't drink either,' Dr Heyden explained. 'And I felt it essential to have patients keep up a high fluid intake and, in those early days, keep a record of what they drank at weekends.' Even as the diet has gradually evolved and been modified, strong emphasis is still placed on a high fluid intake, to flush the kidneys, and a minimum of six glasses of liquid a day is recommended.

When he began the research program, Dr Heyden was working to perfect a diet which would not interfere with people's daily routine - hence so many of his patients were, as Duke employees, on the spot. Then in 1972 came the evolution at Duke. Under the direction of Dr Stulke a diet kitchen was opened in one of the dorms. Meals could now be prepared on the premises strictly in accordance with the diet, and patients could come from far and wide. A new concept had been born. The aim of the program was two-fold: to teach people how to structure their lives so as to achieve their weight-loss goals; and to teach them how to continue the regime back home.

Soon the program was developing rapidly and a bandwagon was rolling. Psychologists were brought in, and they immediately objected to the fasting element of the regime. They called it unstructured non-eating, and felt it was not in the best interests of the patients. With Dr Heyden's agreement it was stopped and the calorie allowance - now increased to 750 a day - was evened out over a seven-day week.

Research into every aspect of the diet continued intensively, and non-stop. At first, for example, there was concern that the diet might be low in potassium. But it was cleared when analysis showed that it never provided less than 3000 mg of potassium a day, against the US minimum daily requirement of 2000 mg.

The diet was also given the all-clear on the matter of sodium content. 'We know that the sodium concentration is less than three grams,' Dr Heyden told me. 'Some people would like it to be less, but we find that a very satisfactory reduction. We have evidence that this is a good restriction of sodium, from the large number of patients who have reduced their blood pressure through this diet.'

Adequate calcium was built into the diet with the allowance of skimmed milk and certain vegetables, and protein - the cornerstone of Dr Heyden's research - was sometimes up to 65 grams a day, five grams more than the government requirement.

In general, the Duke Diet and Fitness Center Diet as it has now evolved, comprises a daily intake of 60 grams of protein, 60 grams of carbohydrate and 25 grams of fat, of which five grams is polyunsaturated.

On this diet which, remember, was devised for grossly overweight patients, Dr Heyden says it is reasonable to expect a permanent cure rate among obese people of 30 per cent. This compares favourably with five per cent only ten years ago, and offers a significant way forward in what Dr Heyden describes as a national epidemic. For obesity in the US has reached epidemic proportions, he acknowledges. About 40 per cent of the population is not of normal weight, and of these, about 25 per cent are grossly overweight.

Dr Heyden has his own personal theory for this alarming figure. He puts it down to the massive numbers of people in the US who, particularly since the 1960s, have quit smoking - a drastic reduction of some 30 per cent.

'This is a phenomenon that is overlooked by our harsh critics in Europe,' he says and points out that in both Europe and Japan it is smoking that is still an epidemic. 'They lament about our obesity and the American life-style, but they don't realize that we have done something much more important for our health. And that is quitting smoking,' he says. Dr Heyden sees a bright way forward. 'We have a much better chance now than we had ten years ago that the weight reduction will be permanent. With all the information and weight reduction programs, it is a national phenomenon. Ten years ago it was an individual decision. Today it is a mass decision. This is a national trend which was absolutely necessary, just as quitting smoking was. Today there is a stigma attached to being a smoker. The obese will soon find themselves stigmatized because of their obesity. In fact, many of them already do feel that way, looking around at all these fit people.'

To sum up: What makes the Duke Diet and Fitness Center Diet such a success is that, one, it is nutritionally sound, approved by the

American Medical Association, meeting all the criteria of the standards set by the government.

Two, it teaches you how to cope with the emotional problems attached to eating behavior, and gives you a personal insight into your own food-and-drink-related problems: something very difficult to achieve without professional help.

Three, you learn to incorporate a fitness program into your daily life. This will play an enormous part in your success in losing the weight and maintaining that loss once you achieve your own goal. And even if your health is already good, your feeling of well-being will certainly improve.

Four, you will have all the tools you need to be a successful weight loser and goal maintainer *in a medically approved manner*, which will drastically improve your health and help you to lead a longer and happier life.

And five, this really is a plan for life, because you simply increase your calories once you reach your goal weight and then, quite naturally and easily, will remain on the program for the rest of your life.

Let Dr Heyden have the last word: 'From whatever viewpoint you look at it, we have looked into all the aspects of the diet and found them compatible with good health and safe weight loss.'

Chapter 1

Personal History

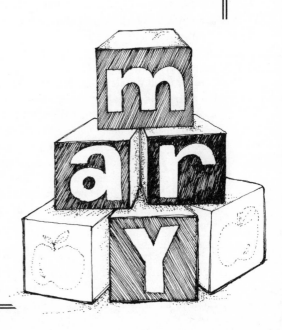

Chapter 1
Personal History

Well, I guess I am just like the rest of you. I love to eat. I was always going to lose weight some day. But for most of my life, this was a decision I was more than happy to put off. I was going to lose weight this year, next year, sometime. But there was no great urgency.

Actually, I was waiting for that magic pill that would save me the trouble. You know, the one the scientists are finally going to come up with so that we fat people can eat all the food we love, take this magic pill and it will dissolve any excess calories our bodies don't need. And there we will all be - beautiful, skinny, healthy and eating anything we want whenever we want.

Failing that, I used to think, the good fairy will appear, wave a magic wand over me, and I will wake up thin and happy. Yet another fantasy I used to have - yes, I have gone to extremes - was that I would be hit by a car while I was crossing the street, be in a painless coma for three months and when I finally woke up I would weigh about one hundred pounds. Then, of course, I would have to eat and eat to get my strength back. Pure heaven, eh?

Now what do all these fantasies have in common? They prove that we fat people want to hand control of our problem over to someone or something else. So the first thing that I and probably you face is that *we are responsible for our problem*. It's not my mother or your husband. We may have problems with these people, but only *you* can control what happens when people or situations stress you out. The only person that you can change is you. There is no magic pill, no fairy Godmother and, with luck, no street accident. What there has to be is real determination, grit and hard work, plus hunger pangs in the beginning. But at the end there is a new you and a thin body and this incredible feeling of accomplishment.

No-one's pretending that it's easy. I've heard it said that if you are an alcoholic you need never have another drink. There are plenty of look-alike and even taste-alike alternatives. But if you are a foodaholic you have to eat to stay alive. So it's a constant temptation.

Not only that, we all live in a food-oriented society. Pick up any magazine today and what's usually on the cover in big black letters? 'New way to lose 10 pounds in 10 days'. Buy the magazine - as you certainly would with a statement like that - and what's on the first page? A new recipe with pictures in living color for a chocolate cake. How can you win?

Our whole culture is based on food. When you are having people over what's the first thing you think about? 'What shall I serve?' It's never, 'What will we talk about?' or 'What color flowers shall I order?' We are a food-based society and we just have to learn to live with it. Those of us who are trying to lose weight and keep it off must be constantly alert to these things. We must be subversive of this whole culture. We must program ourselves to think away from food. For lovely indulgent foodie thoughts lead us straight into temptation. And that's the path we can't take.

I would like to tell you a little about my background, my family, my upbringing, my almost daily battle with my weight problem, and the mind problem that went with it; my achievements, early failures and, at last, the path I finally took to a goal I could attain and hold on to. I feel that if you come with me, you will realize you are not alone and, best of all, you can end up with the same sense of achievement and fulfilment as I have. You will also be able to look yourself in your mirror or a glass window in a shop and love what you see reflected there. And isn't that something?

I was always going to lose weight 'some day'. I had lots of time and life was never going to end. Sounds familiar? When the children grow up, when the marriage straightens out, when Christmas is over, and on and on and on. I was suddenly brought up short by the illness of the sister of a friend of mine. She, the sister, was fifty years old and she had lung cancer. I myself was 48 and it struck home. I was suddenly face to face with my own mortality. It was something I had avoided facing. I was really going to die some day. I didn't have endless time. I could no longer live in a fool's paradise of, 'One day I am going to lose weight, see Europe, a World Series, the Panama Canal.' My future was now. And I'd better get on with it. If I was going to lose weight ever it had better be now.

But let's go back more or less to the beginning for a moment and see where I had come from. Looking back on it, I realize that the feeling of being fat, if not actually being so, goes back a long way with me. You can say I had a distorted body image at a very early age. Can you go way back into your childhood and try and remember the first picture you have of yourself in your mind's eye? I can.

What I come up with is a fat little girl with terribly straight hair and a ribbon which wouldn't stay on, because my hair was so straight. I was six years old and, I felt, the only fat little girl in first grade. I found an old photo not long ago and, to my surprise, there was another child even fatter than I. What in the world made me feel like that at the age of six years? Not only did I think I was very fat (though the picture actually shows that I was no more than chubby), but I also felt tall - which I certainly never was. So even at that tender age I had a very distorted body image.

To make matters worse I had an elder sister who was terribly skinny and even, wouldn't you know, had curly hair! Next to my sister Joanna even Twiggy would have seemed overweight. As I look back and remember those days my most vivid recollections are all food-oriented.

Just to give you a brief idea of how it all started, Joanna had a health problem when she was born and the doctor told my mother not to let her cry. Two years later, Joanna's health was fine but Mother was still spoiling her. Then I came along. So what does a rotten, spoiled two-year-old do to maintain her share of the attention? What makes Mother most anxious of all? That's easy. Food! Since the new baby is good and eats everything, Joanna, even at the tender age of two years, decided she'd quit eating, and that would get her all the attention she wanted. And did it work!

Breakfast times, as we got older, were a nightmare. Joanna wouldn't drink milk. We even had orange milk, ugh! Nor would she eat eggs - or anything else. By the time she had made her protest in various ways, the whole room was a mess and the family was in chaos. And how did I manage to please Mother? By eating and not making a fuss, of course.

So here am I, pleasing everybody by eating everything that's put in front of me. And now Mother looks at me and says, 'Whoa there. You're beginning to get fat!' Now I had some of her attention all to myself. Was I going to give that up? Not on your life!

It is said that there are three factors involved in how we view our bodies. One is physiological, or physical; one is emotional, and one is cultural. Well, by the age of six or seven I knew all about the physiological and emotional factors, I can tell you. And the cultural one is all around us all of the time.

I had short legs and what do you think? When Joanna and I walked to school, she refused to walk along with me. She always strode on ahead and my little fat legs just couldn't keep up. I would shout at her, 'I'm going to tell Mama.' Since she wouldn't wait for me, I would stop off at Rosedale pharmacy and steal Luden's cough drops and a candy bar every morning. At least, I thought I was stealing them. Since we had a charge account there, it was probably being put on our bill all the time. I hope so, anyway.

18

Now for the highly-charged emotional factor. My parents divorced when I was six. Since I considered myself my father's favorite I was really feeling alone and deserted. Somehow I got the idea that it was my fault they separated, and since that was the beginning of my feeling fat, maybe I was somehow punishing myself for whatever I thought I had done. Anyway, I do believe that was the beginning of my body image problem.

Added to that, it was just my luck that my family was even more food-oriented than most. We lived in the Southwest and everyone had a cook, and a fantastic cook at that. My great aunt Bebe, who was older than my grandmother and had no children, invited us to lunch every Saturday. And she always let us plan the menu - pork, corn, chocolate cake, anything. Although she fought being fat all her life, her husband was skinny and she was always pushing food on him, so my own enthusiasm for everything that was put in front of me fitted right into the family pattern. That was one place I could eat all I wanted and brother, I have to tell you that I did! Do you know that at Aunt Bebe's they served the buttered corn so hot they had to pour a jug of cold, sizzling water over it to cool it down. I loved that splattering sound! My sister, of course, true to form, picked at her food as usual, but no-one seemed to notice it at Aunt Bebe's.

It was rather different on Sundays at home, though some of my fondest childhood memories are of summer Sundays at our own house, with a groaning table filled with fried chicken, rice and gravy, fresh corn, salads, a coconut or chocolate cake and home-made ice cream. That was the stuff our family ritual was made of. But it was constantly marred for me by the question that was always on my mother's lips, 'Shall we let Mary have dessert today?' Imagine putting a child at a table staggering under the weight of all that food and then expecting her not to eat! I have questioned her since, and asked her why she was so disturbed about a small child being chubby, and her answer was simply, 'looks'.

Every bit as conflicting were the Friday-night get-togethers at my grandmother's house. Every Friday she had her side of the family and my family for dinner. There was always Aunt Estelle, an example to us all. She had been married and had no children, and then her husband had left her. Family rumour had it that he was driven away because she was so fat. At any rate, at a very early age I got the idea that if you were fat your loved ones left you, so that fat was not a good thing to be. It made you ugly and probably resulted in your being an old maid. So early on I had this really bad feeling about myself, and boy was I confused. Talk about double messages!

On these Friday nights about eight or ten of us sat down to really memorable meals. Huge, delicious dinners, they were - chicken curry, sirloin chili, crown of lamb, peach pies - I can smell it all now. And since Joanna and I were the only grandchildren, we were made much over. But almost more than the array of totally irresistible food, and my grandmother eating whipped cream piled on to bread, the other over-powering thing I remember is my sister being constantly nagged to eat, and me being told not to eat so much. Not that my grandmother set much of an example herself. She never cared how fat she got. She just went out and bought a larger size of corset. She always dressed exquisitely and loved clothes, but being thin did not figure on her list of priorities. And being the person she was, she got away with it.

For me it was different. There was I, under the watchful and critical eye of my mother. To eat or not to eat was always the confusing question. But these were mistakes of the head, not of the heart, and I understand all of this now. Joanna and I have talked over our separate childhood roles endlessly, we each understand the other's viewpoint, and we are the best of friends. But it sure was hard to achieve that sisterly harmony when we played such opposing roles across the dinner table! And of course it all served to confuse me utterly about food, and that confusion stayed with me right into adulthood. This whole business gave food, in my mind, connotations which food should not have. Very emotional connotations. Food was used as reward and punishment, not as a source of body energy and of pure pleasure. I can tell you, you would have had to be a genius to work that one out for yourself.

This question of the image you have of yourself from childhood plays tricks both ways. My sister Joanna, whom I now adore and have long since forgiven for being a thin person with curly hair, has gained weight in later years. But I really believe that she has as hard a time seeing herself as overweight now as I do at realizing I am close to normal weight. And, of course, as we all know, even this image isn't constant. Your day-to-day mood changes affect how you see yourself just as surely as if you were looking in one of those funny mirrors in the amusement park. If I look at myself in the glass on a day when I'm feeling fine, I'll think, 'Boy, I really do look nice.' But the following day, if I'm not feeling good about something, I can look in a mirror and think, 'Gee, but I really am fat.' Same mirror. Same me. No rapid gain in weight. Just a distorted mental body image. It really is hard to hold on to a clear picture of yourself as you actually are.

So, I grew up with this double message. Eat. Don't eat. I realize now, I never really got to control my own eating habits, nor did my sister. Mother took us over as babies, which is appropriate. But she never really knew how to teach us our own control. So that in later life I ate for all sorts of reasons, rarely from hunger for food alone.

I believe that many people have similar backgrounds, which turn food into all sorts of emotional whammies. And if you look back at your own childhood and try and sort out when was food just food, and when was it a weapon, a comfort, a substitute, perhaps you can reach some insight into your present eating habits. At least, that's why I decided to write this book. To help you do just that. Because, chances are these things are still going on. And it sure is hard to fathom them out.

I believe now that a lot of my early eating was an effort to control my life in at least one aspect. Besides the fact - never far from the front of my mind - that I really loved food!

There was just one great period of my life when food was pushed to the back of my mind. As I grew up - I never grew tall - my primary interest in food gave way for just one brief moment to an interest in boys, having dates and going to dances. Through my late teens and early twenties I did not have a single problem with my weight. It was wonderful! I got busy with a job I liked and was totally absorbed in life itself and not, for once, in food. Then, when I was 29, I got married. Next I got pregnant and we moved to London to live. Before I left the States my general practitioner told me to be careful. The hardest weight to lose was the weight gained during pregnancy. Other medical opinions now say that the hardest weight to lose is what they call child-onset obesity. Me, I now had both!

From the time I was three months pregnant I started eating everything I could get my hands on. The food halls at Harrods were just about full enough for me. And how I loved not worrying about my weight going up! It wasn't me, it was our baby, wasn't it? If I had been taller, I tell myself, perhaps my problem wouldn't have been so acute. But as it was, at five-foot-two I was getting squarer by the minute. After - yes, after - our little girl, Bebe, was born, I weighed 180 pounds (12 stone 12lb). And after a massive effort I had just gotten down to 160 pounds (11 stone 6lb) when oops - I was pregnant again. It was only eleven months later.

My husband and I were having problems and this pregnancy was hard on me. The combination of living so far from home, trouble within my marriage and a year-old baby to look after really took its toll. So, what did I turn to but food, food, food. The old standby. And I went up like a balloon.

We went back home when our son was two months old. It was July in Houston, Texas, and the temperature was over 100F (37C) every day. I ate for every reason and as an excuse for everything that was wrong with my life. Don't imagine that I just went out and ate without thinking. I thought a lot about it. But I still ate!

Full of guilty feelings, I went into psychotherapy to try and put my life together. I worked hard on myself in therapy for a very long time. Then, when I got to a certain point in the therapy, I looked at my five-foot-two and 235-pound (that's a cool 16 stone 11lb) outside and realized it no longer looked like the me that was on the inside. I felt good about myself now, and I wanted the outside to match. So began my diet odyssey, an adventure which was to last me for the rest of my life.

Chapter2

Good and Bad Behavior

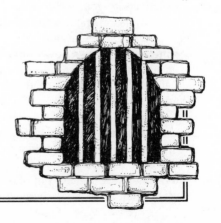

Chapter 2
Good and Bad Behavior

Human behavior is not random, it is motivated by stimuli and by consequence. This sounds very profound, but as I got more into trying to lose my weight it became more and more apparent that my weight and my emotions were all tangled up together. I began to realize that my obesity was a symptom. A symptom, among other things, of how I felt about myself and how I looked at the world.

The picture I have is of people carrying a lot of baggage with them when they become adults. How much baggage you have depends a great deal on what you were saddled with in childhood and during your growing-up years. And I'm not just talking about the obvious excess baggage carried as overweight on the body. I'm talking about extra baggage of the mind, too.

Example: you meet someone named Cynthia and take an instant dislike to this person upon hearing her name. Now why in the world would you do that? Think about it and what do you come up with? It's that snotty little girl you knew in third grade who was a miss goody-two-shoes, teacher's pet and always looked so neat that all the other girls looked like slobs next to her. Her name was Cynthia and everybody hated her. So, whenever you hear that name now, all these years later, it's a conditioned response. Like Pavlov's dogs, but instead of salivating, you find a feeling of dislike arising within you. Unfair, yes. Unreasonable, maybe. Unusual, it certainly is not.

This is just one example of human behavior which is motivated by stimuli, and shows how difficult it can be to recognize and come to terms with. Luckily food-orientated reactions are somewhat easier to define. I find, for instance, that if I am hungry I had better not read my gourmet food magazine. Obviously. Because then I get even more hungry and may well eat something I don't want to eat - or at any rate shouldn't be eating. So, if I want to change my behavior and go on a diet I know I had better avoid the apparent food cues which I know make me want to eat. I'll come later to those food cues that are around us all the time that are not of our own making. It is very important to identify them and look them square in the eye. You can't change your behavior pattern until you can identify these stimuli, both internal and external.

I came from a family which had very rigid ideas about all human emotions. Some were permitted - all the good ones. But most of the 'bad' ones, such as anger, greed, jealousy, nice people 'didn't have'. So I imagine I covered up a lot of emotions with food.

In order to be a successful dieter and to change your eating behavior you have to see positive consequences of your actions. The trouble with dieting is that very often some positive consequences are a long way down the road.

Getting on the scale and seeing a weight loss is a wonderful and positive consequence of your diet. Even better was the day I was in the grocery store and a friend of mine looked at me, then looked away, did a double take and came back and said, 'Hey, Mary, is that you?' Sure it was me, but a new me, and did I feel good that he hadn't at first recognized me.

To my mind - having been a fat person myself for most of my life - one of the most fascinating conundrums in the whole world is why some people are overweight and others are not. Why some people, even in the same family, can eat anything they want and hardly put on an ounce, while others might be eating far less and are obese.

Even now, after all the research, not much is known about the reasons for overweight, other than too many calories are taken in and too few expended. Is it all to do with our glands? Is it hereditary? Can we really blame our great aunt Martha for giving us this tendency to easy weight gain? Or is it - just possibly - something we do to ourselves? There is no doubt that some people, because of their particular metabolism, are much more susceptible to weight gain and, indeed, to the stimulus of food, than others; more of that later. But what it really comes down to, and what we are concerned about here, is that those of us who are overweight simply eat too much. We eat more calories than our bodies burn up in energy. And calories equal fat - and usually in all the wrong places, too.

The only way to lose weight is to eat less, and the only way to do this is to make up your mind to do it. Eating less, once you are on the right path, is comparatively easy. Making up your mind to do it, and sticking to that resolve, is the hardest bit. Which is why this chapter is really the most important in the book, all about how to know your own strengths and weaknesses and how to structure your behavior so that you can make up your mind to restructure your life - and then do it.

The fact is that in order to lose one pound in weight (about 450g) you have to eat 3,500 calories less. 'Three thousand five hundred calories!' I can hear you shriek. 'Why, I bet I don't even eat that many in a week.' I bet you do, and a whole lot more than you think. I know I did, until the answer to the question, 'Who's counting?' was, 'I am, now!'

Okay, let's see. How about breakfast. Oh, you don't eat breakfast, right? How about those two donuts you eat when you get to work - having rushed out without touching a thing: 250 calories each. Or the Danish pastry at coffee break, another 300 calories to add to the total. Then, let's see. Lunch. Because you didn't eat any breakfast (except of course that small 500-calorie snack) you can go all out at lunch. What's that you say? You only go to this place with a salad bar. Well, let me tell you something. A 'salad bar' with half a cup of regular dressing is around 750 calories. And how about this: a ten-inch (25-cm) pizza with topping is 1,100 calories. A piece of apple pie is 350. A double hamburger with cheese is a mighty 600. So, you have the salad bar 'snack' and think you've been so good.

Along about 4 pm you're starving again, so how about some candy to sort of pick up your energy? A one-ounce (25g) chocolate candy bar tots up 150 calories, five cookies add another 250 and a can of coke comes to 150. So far you've eaten about 1,800 calories and you haven't even had dinner!

When you get home you're exhausted, of course, so you figure since you've been so good you'll have a drink. Just a standard measure of vodka or scotch is 75 calories - not too bad, but what about all the 'mixers' we like to put with it? One regular beer is 288, two light beers are 192, and the irresistible handful of peanuts to go with them are 425. When you're drinking and talking 20 potato chips slip down easily, but then so do 250 calories. And ten small crackers with three ounces (75g) of cheese cut up into such small cubes they hardly seem to count do count for rather a lot - another 500 calories to be exact! That little snack that you didn't even notice adds another 617, to bring your calorie total so far to 2,417.

Now, at last, it's dinner time. Three pieces of fried chicken (750), a large order of french fries (500) and a milk shake for dessert (400) and you end your day with 4,067 calories taken in.

And how much energy did you expend? In an office job, if I may say so, *not* very much. So, if you cut down on your daily calorie intake by even 2,000, in one week you're eating 14,000 fewer calories.

Of course, maybe this is an exaggeration. Not everyone, not even those who are 'easy responders' to the stimulus of food, eats 4,700 calories a day. But if you eat 2,000 and expend only 500, you will gain weight.

The point I'm trying to make is this: you must watch and record every mouthful you take in, especially at the beginning of your new program, because almost everything has calories. And you must learn to become acutely aware of what you are eating and why you have been eating it. There's a load of advice on how to monitor and structure exactly what you eat in the Nutrition section.

You must already have decided to lose weight - or why have you bought this book? The next question is, why have you decided to do it? This is important, because it is the reason that drove you to make a start which will keep you going through thick and thin. Perhaps you looked in the mirror one day and finally saw yourself as you really are - fat. Or someone took a picture of you at the family picnic and you came face to face with a shape that you didn't recognize as the real you. Or you caught your husband looking at that cute slim blonde who lives next door. So, you're going to try and get back into a size 10 again.

A word of caution, right at the start. Who are you losing weight for? Your husband? Your lover? Your children? Your friends? Yourself? If it's not the last of these, forget it. If you lose weight for anyone other than you, you are probably going to fail.

Why? Well, it's like this. If you lose weight for your husband, the minute he makes you angry you are going to eat to punish him. You'll get mad. You'll say, 'I'll fix him. I'll go eat something.' And before you know it, there you are, standing at the ice-box pushing a piece of chocolate cake into your mouth. At that moment you might not even really want that piece of cake. But subconsciously you are rebelling against your husband, and what you decided to do for him, and so in it goes. Just to get back at him!

After you've eaten that enormous slice of calories, which goes right against your resolve, of course, comes the depression. And what is depression? It's hostility turned inward. Hostility towards yourself now. Silly, isn't it? So the first thing you must do is make the decision to lose weight for yourself, alone. No-one else. That way you stay in control.

It seems to me that staying in control is one of the biggest problems in weight loss. Most of us who have a weight problem also have problems controlling our lives in general. Everyone who has ever been on a diet knows the feeling. You've been doing really well and suddenly you see a cookie or a candy bar or a hunk of cheese or whatever, and wham! You've grabbed it and swallowed it almost without noticing, in direct opposition to your weight-loss goal. You went 'out of control'. And why did you do this? You weren't suddenly any hungrier then than you were before, yet one minute you had the will to resist and the next, you didn't. Why? There doesn't seem to be any real excuse. If there is one thing we should have total control over, it is what actually goes into our mouths.

There may be a load of deep psychological reasons for this. But for me the main answer was that I used to put everyone else's needs before my own. I hadn't learned how to put a fence around myself and save a small space just for me, where I was the most important one. It's like putting a boundary around your house to keep your property uninvaded. Everyone must set boundaries, beyond which people must not encroach. Like the place in your heart where only you can be, your personhood needs boundaries also. If you don't set these limits, if you give everyone else's needs and wants priority over your own, then I have to tell you that you are definitely not in control. And it's when other people's demands encroach on your own that you are likely to eat.

Another thing I have learned is that you really have to like yourself enough to lose weight and keep it off. You have to love yourself enough to think you deserve a beautiful body. That takes a lot of self-love, which we fatties are many times hard pressed to come up with. It took me most of my life to realize that as a child I was led to believe that a lot of myself was bad, because I didn't measure up to someone else's idea of what beautiful was. In the eye of the beholder, indeed! I was never allowed to control my own appetite. Someone else told me when I was hungry and when I was full. I never developed my own control. So rigid was that parental control over my body that the only way I could rebel was to eat what I wanted when I wanted. The problem was, I never felt full. I know now that what I was trying to fill up on was love. Food is used extensively in our society as a substitute for love. The TV ad says, 'Put a little love in his lunchbox,' and what does that mean? Candy. Isn't that awful? Learning to distinguish between emotional hunger and real hunger is not easy when you've always mixed them up.

Finding out why you eat, when you eat, why you binge is one of the hardest things. It takes a lot of self-analysis and more honesty than a lot of us can muster. Behaviorists have found out that people who are overweight react more to food cues than others. For instance, if a thin person and a fat person had dinner together and then sat down and watched all those gooey food ads on the TV, the thin person wouldn't react at all, because he would be feeling full. But the fat person has to take care. He would forget all about the meal he had just eaten, and he'd be wanting that food that's coming up on the screen in front of him.

And let's face it, that's just what the TV ads are all about. Their job is to make us feel hungry even when we're not, to break down our resistance to food we don't need and shouldn't be having. Who can watch that hamburger frying and being put together in vivid color while these insistent TV voices keep asking, 'Aren't you hungry? Aren't you hungry for a burger now?' I wasn't, but I sure am now!

This is something you've got to learn about yourself. If you are more sensitive to food cues, one of the easy responders, you've got to know what to do about it when those cakes, burgers and ice cream come on the TV. Get up and turn it off, that's the best thing to do, because you know you're over-sensitive. If there is someone else in the room who wants to go right on watching, then you're going to have to get up and walk out of the room. And not straight to the ice-box, either!

It's a tough lesson to learn. The whole of our culture is based on food, right from the time we are young. Ask any kindergarten child what Thanksgiving is and I'll bet his answer will be, 'Turkey day'. Talk to a friend who's just come back from a trip and sure enough, the first thing you ask is, 'What was the food like?' We Americans, and most of the people in all the other developed countries of the world, I guess, are absolutely wrapped up in food. Foreigners probably think that whenever we get together we talk about money mostly. Wrong - it's food.

We talk a lot about dieting too - we sure need to. In fact, a world-famous journalist recently said - with only a small degree of journalistic licence - that we buy only two kinds of books in the US, those that show you how to prepare and cook the most delicious food, and those that tell you how to take off the weight afterwards! That's about right, but - sorry for the commercial! - this book does both. It shows you how to prepare and cook the most delicious but low-calorie food, and it shows you how to resist all the other kinds. For this is not a diet, it's a life program, and it begins right there in your head. Obviously making up your mind to lose weight is the single most important step you'll ever take towards shaping up the new you. This book is the key to that resolve.

Now, when are you going to start? Monday? We all start our diets on Monday. I really knew I was in earnest when I started my diet on a Thursday. There is a wonderful poem by Judith Viorst entitled 'Starting on Monday' which says it all. Don't wait until Monday. *Do it today.* Let's be honest. There is never the ideal time. You will always be able to find an excuse not to start now if you want one. You have a dinner party coming up. You're going to a wedding or a barmitzvah. Thanksgiving, Hallowe'en, Christmas is coming. There'll be candies around for the kids. Extra goodies all over the house and of course extra temptation. But that's the point. If you're really in earnest you can start on the day you're going out to dinner, sampling just a little of everything and really enjoying the sensations of flavor.

What I call your Mind Set is very important. If you are now in earnest, losing weight has to be a top priority in your life. Make up your mind here and now that anything which stands in the way of your weight loss *will not be tolerated.* You don't have to announce to all and sundry that you are dieting - though some people find it easier to stick to their regime if they have told others. It's kind of losing face if you then go back on your word. But in any case, keep this new resolve always in the front of your mind.

And how to do this? Those of you who have ever closely observed cats may have noticed what is called their 'alternative behavior'. When you scold your cat or speak loudly to it, or if it gets frightened, it will begin to wash itself. This is a clever trick to distract your mind from whatever the cat did in the first place to displease you, and presumably to take the cat's own mind off the uncomfortable feeling he has that all is not well between you. Good thinking!

When you are trying to lose weight, you need not one but many alternative behaviors, ways to trick yourself away from the forbidden foods, the downward path. You have to put your personal computer on to *think thin*. And then when you are tempted by the wrong foods you can have the will to resist. Take boredom, for example. What do most people do when they are bored? If we can't find anything else to occupy our minds most of us start thinking about food. And not only thinking, either!

When you start getting this all-too-familiar craving for food, the best thing you can do is to get out of the house - quickly. If you really are tied to the house and can't get away for a bit, find something constructive to do with your hands. I used to pick up a piece of needlepoint. For one thing it kept my mind and my hands occupied, and of course you always tend to say, 'I'll wait until I get to the end of this row before getting up and getting something.' And hopefully by then the feeling will have worn off! Another thing, when I was doing a piece of fine work I didn't even want to eat a chocolate bar and risk getting a smudge all over my neat, painstaking work. Better still, turn on the radio or put on a cassette - and dance. The exercise of both the mind and the body will be good for you. It is now a proven fact that light exercise such as fast walking and, yes, dancing will burn off more calories than was once thought to be the case.

If you do have the opportunity, go outdoors for a bit. As soon as you open your door and step outside the desire for food will lessen, I promise you. Just movement and changing your environment eases your feelings of hunger. Now you can go and work in the garden, go for a walk, phone up a friend and ask if you can go to her house (but tell her why; then she won't try to feed you!), take the children to the park, get in the car, go to a movie, go to the town and look in the shop windows, whatever takes your fancy. If you still feel hungry, then just *feel* hungry. You will *not* starve to death until supper. Feeling hungry means losing weight. Make friends with your hunger.

Shop for your new wardrobe in a size which you want to be when you reach your goal. There's no better incentive to weight loss than having a new dress or suit in the wardrobe which you can't yet get into.

If you feel that's going a bit too far, shop in your mind, from your head to your toes. Go into the stores and look at all the size 10s, or 8s, or even 6s. Whatever your goal size is. Pick out the dress, the coat, the hat, the shoes, the whole thing. By the time you've done this, you'll have got over the feeling that you want to eat something forbidden. That all seemed such a long time ago, you had forgotten all about it, hadn't you?

I was telling someone about this particular suggestion for alternative behavior and do you know the first thing she said? 'But I couldn't do that, no way. The movies is the very place where I do snack. Candies, cookies, cola drinks, I have to have them all.' Well, you don't have to have them, of course. But if you are used to snacking in the movies, take a bag of celery and pepper sticks with you the first few times. They're not all that anti-social - they don't sound any louder than popcorn! And take a diet drink also. Then quickly cut down on the amount you take, until you take nothing with you but an interest in what's on the screen.

If you are a snacker and between-meal eater, it's a habit you need to do away with, at home, in the movies, wherever you are. I read somewhere that you can break any habit in three weeks. Cut out all snacks for that time and you will probably be cured for all time. If you can't cure yourself, have raw vegetables ready and chilled in the fridge so that when you open the door, that's the first thing you see. Not that piece of cake left over from yesterday's coffee party. That's fatal.

So many people I have talked to have this hang-up about left-over food. When I was a child I was told that I must eat up all the food on my plate because of the starving Armenians. That's when I wasn't being told, of course, whoa, Mary, you're putting on weight! Friends in the UK tell me that they had to clean up every last bit of food because of the starving people in China. No-one ever thought to explain to the children what difference it would make to those less fortunate than ourselves whether we ate the food on our plates or not. I used to spend a long time wondering how my scraps were ever going to get to Armenia and still be in a fit state to be eaten. Or why, as they needed them so much more than I did, I wasn't being encouraged to put some food by for them. It was just another of life's confusing food-oriented problems when I was a child.

However, it made a lasting impression on me, and on so many more people I know. It took me many years before I could actually bring myself to waste food. To make an omelet with three egg whites and throw the yolks down the waste-disposer in the sink. I didn't want them. The Armenians weren't ever going to get them, so out they went.

When I began dieting seriously, and was only just beginning to learn how to cope with the many day-to-day temptations, I wouldn't ever clear the table. I'd get the kids to do it for me. I couldn't bear to do it myself - all that food! Then I'd go out into the kitchen to cope with the dishes once the food was out of sight. Otherwise that morsel of pie that was left would really get me. I'd tell the kids to throw it down the sink, put it in the garbage can, anything, but get it out of my sight. I hate waste as much anybody, I still do, but what's the point of eating food you don't want? I've stood there at the fridge door, I can tell you, and eaten a plate of cold spaghetti. Almost half a lemon meringue pie. I'd think, 'Oh well, we're going out tonight. I'd better do it a favor and finish it up. Just this once, of course.' But we really have to get out of this 'waste not, want not' way of thinking. 'Waist not' is what it should be. This food is empty calories anyway, and sure would be going to waste as great lumps of fat on your body!

I've always had this problem with food in the ice-box. If I know there's something really wonderful in there, and I'm in the house, it seems to call out to me. But if I get up and go into the garden or upstairs, I don't hear it. Try that. That way, you are distancing yourself from the food, and the temptation. People who are overweight have to fool themselves constantly with little tricks. It is these tricks which make all the difference between being able to resist temptation and giving in to it - just one more time.

There comes a time when you really do have to remember that you're dieting for yourself, and no-one else. Your loved-one, trying to be kind, and knowing the sacrifices you are making, says, 'Oh come on, try a piece of this. Just once won't matter.' Oh yes it will, and now you know it. One of the hardest problems I used to have was when I had come back from a course at the Duke Diet and Fitness Center and my husband, who is very interested in wine, would bring out a special bottle he had been saving to welcome me - the new me - home. Now this is difficult. You might know that wine can be your downfall, and one glass will lead to two, and then your inhibitions are weakened, and you could eat something not on your program at all.

So how to handle this without hurting your husband's feelings? Do you get angry - as I might have done at one time - and yell something like, 'How could you do this to me? You're just trying to destroy all I've done,' and burst into tears? That's aggressive behavior. Or do you smile, drink the wine and loathe your husband, promising yourself you'll get even with him? That's passive aggressive, and you don't do that either. You say something like, 'How sweet of you to think of me in this way. You know how much I love wine. But could we save it for another time, when I feel I can handle it better? I'm not too sure of myself yet. But thank you anyway.' That's assertive and mostly it works very well. No wine. And definitely no hurt feelings!

In this respect you will have to learn - and it can be hard - to put your own priority before that of everyone, even the children, even when they complain that sweets have disappeared from the house. Tell them to eat their sweets out of the house, or out of your sight. You just can't do with unnecessary temptation. And let's face it, who can resist a candy a child holds out so lovingly?

Sometimes your weight-loss program just does have to affect others in the family. In our household nuts loomed up as a large obstacle standing in the way of my goal. We always had a large jar of mixed nuts on the bar, and my husband liked to have a handful when he sat down with a drink after coming in from the office. I was convinced all the time that I was buying them for him. But every time I passed the bar I had a handful of those nuts, too, so I quit buying them. I said to myself he doesn't need them, for sure I don't need them, so I just won't buy them. It's tough. But altering your way of life is tough. Do you know once when he was going away on a business trip he had the nerve to buy some nuts before he went, and fill up that jar with them. He didn't do it on purpose, but every time I went by I had to look at them. There got to be less in the jar every day, of course. It's a great deal easier to resist temptation if it isn't there in front of your eyes!

Social behavior comes into your new program more than you might think. Be on the look-out for fat friends who do not have your will to survive the diet program, and others who have never had to think about their own weight, and therefore think the whole thing is a lot of fuss about nothing. Sure as anything, some of them will be hoping you'll fail. You must be strong. And being strong means risking friendships and putting up with loud complaints. Nothing wonderful ever comes easy. The oyster puts up with a lot of irritation with that grain of sand before a pearl appears! Your 'pearl' is going to be walking into a regular store and buying a normal size dress. Your pearl is going to be looking in the mirror at yourself from the neck down - not only from the neck up as you have before.

Example: you are going out to dinner at a friend's house and your resolve is still rather new and tender. Call up and ask for the menu. Explain to your host or hostess that you have allergic reactions to certain foods. This is the absolute truth. You break out in fat if you eat certain things! If you broke out in hives your hostess would be very sympathetic. The fact that you break out in fat should be no less important either to her or to you.

'It's not what you eat, it's the way that you eat it,' could be one of the best slogans for sticking to your diet program. For I found that how I ate my food controlled what I ate. And how I ate definitely became one of the modes of alternative behavior I adopted. We have already seen that many of us don't really count, calorie-wise, the food we sneak from the ice-box, snatch from the jar in passing, eat standing up at the kitchen table. But those calories add up just like any others. Even faster, actually!

Now I've got lots of ideas to fight this quick, stolen snacking. And I believe this theory, which is very strongly built into the Duke program, that it is absolutely vital that you are acutely aware of everything you eat. We kid ourselves that food we have not noticed ourselves eating doesn't count because we cannot clearly remember what it was. Who're you kidding? Now here's the trick. Never eat anything standing up. Don't watch television while you eat. The chances are that your mind will be more on the TV program than on your eating program. And which is more important to you? Don't read a paper or magazine while you're eating, not even if you're in a restaurant alone. It's far more interesting to watch the people going by! Because if you have been reading throughout the meal the chances are that you have put the food into your mouth, swallowed it and not savored it or even tasted it at all. And certainly not calculated the calories.

Eat in style. Even if you are eating alone. Always set the table properly. Put out a place mat or a cloth. Get out your best china and cutlery. Make an occasion of it. And be sure to give yourself a one-size-smaller plate. This is another trick to fool the eye. A diet-sized portion on a smaller plate looks like a generous helping. On a large dinner plate it still looks like a diet-sized portion!

Bear in mind that as you will actually be eating less food in future, it is all the more important - vitally important - to enjoy it. Really savor your food. Concentrate on what it feels like and tastes like in your mouth. Chew it slowly and carefully - some people say you should chew each mouthful of food at least ten times before swallowing it - so that you are conscious in every way of what you have eaten.

This is where fast eaters have a lot of homework to do. Fast eating is out! If you are in the habit of shovelling in your food as quickly as you can and then getting on with the next thing - the hallmark of a busy person - stop! There are lots of things you can do to slow yourself down. The American already has one of the answers. He cuts his meat, puts his knife down, transfers his fork to his right hand, and then picks it up and eats. It's going to take you twice as long like that. I was taught that the right thing to do is not to cut up all your meat at one time, that's 'not done'. You cut one piece of meat, pick up a fork, eat the meat, put the fork down again. Of course the English think this is very funny because it is such a waste of time. But if you are dieting and trying to gain the maximum pleasure from a smaller amount of food, this is a tremendous help. If you use a knife and fork in the regular way, get into the habit of putting them down between every mouthful. Put them right down on your plate and take your hands away. Don't do as so many fast eaters do - always have the next forkful of food ready to put into your mouth as soon as you have finished the last one. That's the sure path to forgetting you ever had anything to eat, and therefore not feeling satisfied in any way at all.

Another good trick, a bit extreme perhaps, is to eat only with chopsticks - especially if you're not very adept with them. For quite a time I ate most of my food with lacquered chopsticks, and I can tell you it's not easy to eat without knowing it if you have to grip everything between two thin, slippery sticks. You just have to eat slowly because you are going to take up very small amounts, and it's going to be a real business to eat anything at all. Until you are sure of your resolve, try it. Eat absolutely everything with chopsticks. Peas. Potatoes. Salad. You will soon find that you automatically cut down on your intake and extend the time it takes you to eat it. And that way the message will get to your brain that you feel full and have eaten enough.

Have you realized that all this - finding ways to enjoy your food even more - is the real secret to success? How many diets have you started and then given up in disgust or despair after a few days? It could be that the food was so deadly dull, that lettuce leaf and half a grapefruit that you ate standing up at the filing cabinet or in the kitchen, that you thought there was no longer any fun in eating. My solution is this. Eat less. Eat wisely. But eat it slowly and enjoy every morsel. There's a whole load of fun in that, and a great deal of satisfaction.

In other words, change your behavior. Reprogram your personal computer - *your mind*. Change the way you look at, manage and think about food. Take charge of your body and your appetite. Refuse to let it take charge of you any longer. Changing your behavior will change your life and ultimately change your body, and give you the best of feelings about yourself. You've won the hardest battle of all: taking charge of your life and your goals.

Promoting Good Health

Chapter 3
Promoting Good Health

Everyone who decides to go on to a weight-loss program does so for a specific reason. For many of us the thing that finally tipped the scales (sorry!) in favor of starting now is a cosmetic, or 'mind' reason. You know, you catch a glimpse of yourself in a store window and hardly recognize that tubby little frame as your own. You might suddenly get the urge to buy some new clothes, and be determined to look like a model in them; want to be more attractive to your partner; attract admiring glances the way you used to or - most important -desperately want to feel a whole lot better about yourself. As I have already stressed, you are and always will be the most important person in your life, and you alone are the person you should be losing weight for.

That said, the best possible reason for deciding to lose weight is for the sake of your health both now and in the future. Being moderately over-weight does not present much of a health risk, and most of us can handle weighing, say, 10 per cent more than we should.

Obesity, on the other hand, contributes to frightening list of health problems, coronary heart disease, high blood pressure, diabetes, elevated blood chloresterol, arthritis, and even certain kinds of cancer among them. And as, let's face it, obesity is only over-weight several stops down the line, it as well to recognize what it is and just what it could do to your life and your health. You won't ever need convincing that prevention is better than cure.

Dr Sigrid Nelius, who has been in charge of the medical department at the Duke Diet and Fitness Center since it was formed, stresses that weight-control and weight-loss together are one of the most significant forms of general preventive medicine. Although no-one and nothing can guarantee any of us a life free from disease or illness of any kind, we should do everything in our power to lower the odds. And taking care of our weight is a very big step in the right direction.

Think of it this way. Dr Nelius likens taking sensible steps to achieve and maintain a normal weight pattern to wearing a seat-belt when you climb into the driving seat of an automobile. Letting your weight race ahead without check, she says, is like driving fast along a busy freeway without putting on your seat-belt.

People who would do that (risking breaking the law in Britain) may or may not be the same ones who will eat greasy bacon and eggs every day, uncaring about the amount of animal fat and the effect on their blood cholesterol levels. Playing Russian roulette, I call it, with the gun barrels loaded with bullets of fat. That's not my game. And since you have bought this book, I daresay it isn't yours, either!

Statistics can be boring. That's when they are not positively alarming. Before you slip your mind into neutral I ask you just to take a look at these figures. In the United States now it is estimated that one-quarter of the adult male population and one-half of the adult female population is 10 per cent over-weight. That alone may not be too earth-shattering, but going on from there we find that 14 per cent of men and 24 per cent of women are at least 20 per cent over-weight, and some of them very much more than that.

Further - and this will shatter you in these days of apparent health and fitness awareness - 10 per cent of the children in the United States are over-weight, 80 per cent of those fat children will become fat adults and about 18 per cent of those children who are thin now will grow into over-weight adults. And who is responsible for this state of affairs? We are, the parents. Research has shown that children of obese parents are more likely than others to become obese, not through heredity alone - we can't blame it on that - but through wrongful eating habits.

It is alarming. Recent studies show that paediatricians all over the United States are seeing more and more children under the age of five - think of that - who are obese. The same studies also show that early-onset obesity is more likely to lead to cardio-vascular disease in later life; boys who have this early childhood obesity are more likely than girls to end up with coronary heart disease.

Did I say that you are the most important person in your life? Yes. But all those of us who have the responsibility for shaping our children's eating pattern have a very heavy responsibility indeed. If you follow this healthy Duke diet to reduce and then maintain your own weight, you can be completely confident that these same foods (in greater quantity) are the best insurance policy for the health of the rest of the family.

When exactly does excessive weight become what is medically defined as obesity? Obesity is said to exist when fat represents 25 per cent of the total body weight in adult males and 30 per cent in adult females, and when one is 20 per cent over ideal body weight. This is set out in accepted life insurance tables which show how much you should weigh according to your height and body frame . Looking at the tables with columns setting out the recommended weight for people with large, medium and small frames - well, we have all been there, haven't we, convincing ourselves that of course we have a large frame. What else?

The fact is that you cannot really argue with these tables. Believe me, no-one knows more about your life expectancy and how your weight affects it than the people who calculate the premium on a policy to insure your life. Obesity has now been officially classified as a disease by US insurance carriers, and it is at epidemic proportion.

I tell you, there's no end to the advantages you enjoy when you cut down your weight. I found this out, when the premium I had been quoted on a large life-insurance policy was drastically cut later, in direct ratio to my weight-loss.

Doctors are constantly reminding us that the single biggest cause of premature death in the Western world is coronary heart disease. That is the plain truth. The encouraging fact is that of the ten identified risk factors, seven of them are wholly or partly in our own control (the other three, heredity, age and gender, we are stuck with!).

Looked at in this light, the Duke program has much to offer in the seven deadly sins we can control, which are obesity, a high level of cholesterol, high blood pressure (hyper-tension) diabetes, high uric acid, inactivity and cigarette smoking.

The whole Duke program is geared to general good health; not just the diet, but the behavior section that helps you to stick to your resolve and the exercise element that helps to refresh both mind and body. Follow the program as a whole and you will lay the best possible foundations for a healthy future.

Even if you have only 10 to 15 pounds to lose now, it is as well to know the medical risks one faces by crossing the bridge from overweight to obesity. This can all too easily happen as we grow older. One's ability to metabolize food naturally slows down with age. And so, if we continue to eat the same amount, it follows that we must step up the exercise program to avoid gaining weight.

Gradually increase the amount of exercise you take, yes, but do not make the mistake of drastically cutting down your calorie allowance. That's logical thinking gone mad. Some people think that if they lose a certain amount of weight on a 750-calorie program they will lose more weight, and faster, on a reduction to, say, 500 calories. Not so! In fact, such a reduction is a danger to health. Below an intake of around 700-750 calories the body loses not only fat but lean tissue.

And even at this recommended low calorie level, the body might be short of vitamins, so it is recommended to take one multi-vitamin tablet a day to supplement.

The medical facts may not make exciting reading but as Dr Nelius says, to ignore them is to put your head in the sands and let your health go out of control.

To take account of the facts and resolve to develop a healthy life-style is to lift up your face to a bright future. That's what the Duke program and this book is all about. We're all in it together, shouting for your success.

Chapter 4

The Nutritional Balance

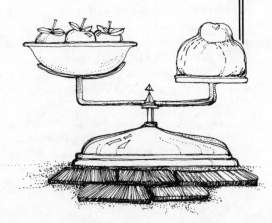

Chapter4
The Nutritional Balance

Isn't it awful how attitudes you formed when you were young stay with you for a greater part of your life? Remember in school how you always fell asleep when it was time to learn about nutrition? I did, anyway. The very name of the class had a mesmerizing effect on me. And as a rule the teacher was a prim little lady with a well-scrubbed face and neat little gestures. But the worst was her voice! It was a complete monotone, and served to make a dull lecture even duller. Who cared about the four food groups? Not us. We liked pizza and hamburgers and ice cream. And, in my case, continued to like them for far too long!

It was many, many years later, when I first attended one of Linda Janick's lectures at the Duke Diet and Fitness Center in fact, before I discovered what a fascinating subject nutrition could be. Linda heads the nutrition department and is not only extremely knowledgable, but also very caring and concerned. She understands that overweight people love everything to do with food, food talk, food pictures, food preparation, and above all eating. And she points out right away what not many people realize - that this obsession with food can be a real asset when you decide to go on a weight-loss program. You can have a great deal of fun, adapting your own favorite recipes into calorie-reduced ones. Fun substituting 'legal' ingredients for fattening ones, and presenting diet food in such a way that it is completely irresistible. Boy, when people start telling me that nutrition can be fun and that diet food really is delicious, I won't fall asleep in their lecture, ever!

The first thing Linda asks patients at the Duke Center - and the first question you should ask yourselves at home - is what your individual eating patterns are. It goes almost without saying that if a person has a weight problem, they have a problem regularizing their meals. 'Afternoon eating, meal skipping, snacking, night eating - these are the most standard occurences we find. On a diet, off a diet; strong diet resolve in the morning, gone by the evening' - Linda says she has heard it all!

Make an honest assessment of your own eating pattern, and resolve here and now to smooth it out. All dieticians agree - and after many false starts, I eventually came round to their way of thinking - that it is important to regularize on three meals a day, at least at first. Planned snacking, if you must, can come later. No skipping breakfast, no matter how late you get up in the morning; no skipping lunch, even if you do want to spend the time window-shopping; and no cutting out one meal to make up for a splurge on another.

I used to be one of the worst, forever skipping breakfast - no time to stop, didn't fancy anything, the usual excuses. I have changed completely now. I've worked out a variety of 150-calorie meals that are really worth getting up for. Now my breakfast can be cereal and fruit, either hot or cold, egg whites fixed like fried eggs (one of my special favorites) and cottage cheese. Quite a treat. An average breakfast calculates like this: 2 egg whites, 30 calories; 1 small box of cereal, 35 calories; half a banana, 45; one-eighth cup low-fat cottage cheese, 25; one-quarter cup skimmed milk, 22. It all adds up to 157 calories, and I've had three courses!

It really is true - for those of you who need convincing - that breakfast is the most important meal of the day. Assuming that you're not a secret night-eater, and haven't eaten anything since bedtime, the blood sugar is at its lowest level when you wake up. The body is then in urgent need of refuelling to give you the energy you need to get through the day.

Let's remind ourselves that that's what a calorie is - energy. One calorie is, very simply, a measure of the energy-producing value of the food. After a meal, the energy produced by the calories consumed is released and used by our bodies for any and all activities. A limit of around 150 calories is reckoned to be all you need to get your day off to a vigorous start, though children and people doing heavy physical work need more.

What energy you don't use, after breakfast and every other meal, is stored in the body for use later - as fat. If later never comes, we become plump little people with too much stored fat - and, contrarily, no energy.

The Duke diet really hammers home the importance of a regular eating pattern. Not only that, the importance of imposing that amount of discipline on yourself. By preparing or taking meals at more or less the same time each day, instead of grabbing a snack on the way through the kitchen, you immediately begin to break the old patterns and institute one which will help you in your weight-loss goals.

Suddenly, just what you eat and when you eat it begins to make sense.

Make a start in shaping your own eating pattern - now. Take a piece of paper and list all the problems you feel you have concerning meals. Do you work and have to take your lunch with you, or get involved day after day in the so-called business-man's lunch? Are you a night-eater, sneaking down to the ice-box when the rest of the family have gone to bed? Do you eat unconsciously while watching television? Be honest with yourself and write it down. All you have to do is identify your problem. We're here to help you solve it. We have ideas for what to take in your little brown lunch bag - and just as important, when to take one - advice on what to choose from a restaurant menu, and heartfelt understanding of how and why some of those cranky eating habits get a hold of people.

Now you have decided that it really is time to do something about losing that 10, 15, 20 or even more pounds, take heart. The one big plus that this program has over all others is that the food you will eat tastes good, and will satisfy you. It might even be the first diet you have ever tried, cross your heart, that applies to. Because of this, believe me, you will find it easy to stay with this program until you reach your goal weight and right on after that. Most diets fail eventually because the food was dull and you couldn't face another minute without something you enjoyed. But not this one!

As always when you are planning to do something positive about your weight, check first with your doctor. This diet is nutritionally sound, but it is always advisable to get his okay for you personally to go ahead.

I have to tell you that once Linda explained the double purpose of including foods from the four groups to provide properly balanced meals, I really began to take notice. With a careful selection from milk and milk products; meat, eggs, fish and poultry; green and yellow vegetables and fruit, and bread, cereals and whole grains, the meals are not only nutritionally correct, they are good and varied. And that's what keeps even the most reluctant dieter cheerfully on course. So many fad diets, and others that claim to be quite serious, ignore this factor completely. Who wants to be faced by a plate of the same one or two food groups day after depressing day? I've been down this road too many times before!

Okay, so you've got the four food groups to choose from and, at the beginning of your weight-loss program, 750 calories to spend. At Duke the calories are divided up to provide 150 for breakfast, 150 for lunch and 450 for dinner. Folks who prefer to eat their main meal during the day can obviously switch the last two. That's the sum total of your expenditure for the first four weeks; after that you can increase your spending, or your calorie intake, gradually.

Talking about 'spending', Linda teaches a system of using calories like you would money. For the first four weeks you are on a budget of 750 dollars, or pounds in the UK. It's a pretty tight budget in calorie terms, but think of it as cash and you begin to feel quite rich. I told you this diet was fun! At the end of that vital first month, if you have reached the weight-loss goal you set yourself, you can say an old aunt died and left you money, and you can add that into your budget. Even if you have not reached your goal weight, after four weeks you should raise your budget by 200-250 dollars, or pounds, or calories. It's a bonanza!

Experience has shown that the make-up of this diet, 60 grams of protein, 60 grams, of carbohydrate and 25-30 grams of fat, is the best recipe for health and for successful weight-loss and maintenance.

Another big factor is that the diet as it is practised at the Duke Center, and set out in the following recipes, is very low in salt, providing up to just 2,000 mg per day. When you realize that most people normally eat between 10,000 and 15,000 mg per day, you can see that this is a vey significant change.

Why is it such a good idea? First, going on what is virtually a salt-free diet (though it more than meets the body's needs) helps you achieve a positive weight-loss sooner. You will get a great deal of satisfaction out of watching the scales plummet - who doesn't? A lot of this early weight-loss will be water. And strangely enough, the more water you drink, the more weight you will lose at first. Eight eight-fluid-ounce (225-ml) glasses of water a day is what's recommended. It sounds a lot, but if you can manage to drink this amount, and at the same time follow the menu plan exactly, you will be amazed at how much weight you lose. And how much time you will spend in the bathroom!

Keeping to a low sodium intake means making a positive choice. Cut out all added salt - never, never put any on the table - and choose low-sodium products. The natural salt in the foods you eat will provide just about the right amount - thankfully, no-one's asking you to sit there and count each separate grain of salt each day! This low-salt diet has another great health bonus - it often lowers blood pressure and relieves hyper-tension, which far too many of us suffer from.

Practically giving up salt overnight does, I have to admit, come as something of a shock, that first week. It sure does affect your taste buds, and that's the idea. It's meant to. The food tastes unfamiliar, and you don't have quite the same craving for it that you would have, if it tasted 'normal'. And no. You don't reach for the salt. That's cheating! Even though the recipes we have devised for you (some are Duke Center specials, some are my own) are pepped up with herbs and sodium-free spices, there's no denying that at first, the food tastes very,

very bland. Then suddenly, without the usual masking flavor of salt, you realize that what you are actually tasting is the food itself. I remember my first salt-free week taught me an important lesson: that pre viously I had been eating to quiet my hunger, not for the enjoy ment of the food itself. This helped me to understand Dr Nelius's advice, 'Eat to live, don't live to eat'.

It is important to realize, too, that at the beginning of the diet there are certain phases you will go through; recognize those and expect to have to make quite a bit of adjustment. As I said, nothing worthwhile ever came easy!

From day one, set your sights on the end of that first week, not on tomorrow. That's important. Miracles don't happen overnight. You know the salt-free food will taste different. You know you will be starting to lose weight, if not immediately then very soon. By the end of the first week you can begin to see the positive results of your weight-loss, and that will give your incentive a real boost. Just when it needs it.

During the second week, you will become used to the taste of the 'new' food, and you will feel more satisfied. I don't say that you won't ever fantasize about food and find it very, very hard not to eat some-thing which is not on your program: you will. But hold firm, because I assure you that, too, will pass! By now, too, much of your 'stomach hunger' and even some of your emotional hunger will be gone. Life gets easier, I promise!

Into week three, and you will feel a great exhilaration because you have succeeded in your resolve for this long. That alone gives you a much-needed boost. You may still occasionally long for some of your old favorite foods, but the desire to go off the program will be greatly lessened.

I found that by the fourth week, those tantalizing fantasies were gone, and no-one on earth would have managed to pry my mouth open to make me eat something that was not on the program. I had begun to control - and even save - my own life! By now of course you can identify the changes in your body - pants loose, shirt getting bigger around the neck and not pulling so tightly on the buttons, stomach smaller - all those things directly related to the changes in your eating pattern. You just wonder why you didn't do it years before!

Choice is the very enemy, the devil, of everyone going on a diet. That's why we have given you a complete four-week menu plan. Stick to it in detail. Don't go to the food store, look along the shelves and try to decide on alternatives. That's the slippery road home!

What we have done is to build a wide choice into the menus. This plan doesn't say only blueberries, or only strawberries, or apples or bananas. It says one half-cup of fruit. This satisfies the nutritional needs as well as the esthetic needs of each individual. You have a yearning to eat strawberries from the time the first berries appear to the very last ones to be picked? You go right ahead and spoil yourself. You prefer the variety of flavor, color and shapes of a mixed fruit salad? Feel free! The menus provide choice, but structured choice, which makes it easy for you to pick your favorite food without going off the rails. I call that real friendly!

Once you have got through that crucial four-week period, and by the time you have reached your goal weight and are on the 'maintenance' program, you can start 'spending' more. You will no longer be on such a tight budget, but can add what I call discretionary income. By now you will be reassured from your own experience that the basic diet is both nutritionally sound and satisfying. But who isn't ready for a bit of a spending spree?

You can begin by adding a little more of the structured foods you have been eating, slightly increasing the portion size. And once in a while, you can add one of those foods that are special to you, and you have been denying yourself. Use this discretionary income with discretion! Don't get carried away. But it is important, for your mind's sake, to feel there is nothing you cannot eat at one time or another - even a piece of chocolate cake. In fact, going into the diet you need to say, 'I can eat a piece of chocolate cake once in a while. It's just that I can't eat it every day.' If you say to yourself that you can never have whatever is your favorite food again, you are doomed from the start.

This is where keeping your food diary comes in useful. Going on a calorie spending spree is like any other. One splurge leads to another. You've had one donut. One or two. What's the difference? A lot in calorie terms, as you will see if it is written down in your book and staring you in the face. Writing down everything you eat, and especially the discretionary treats, leaves you no excuse. If your weight isn't doing what it should, all the evidence is there in your book, and you know just why.

Keep to the basic diet for four weeks and you will have built the foundation of an eating plan for the rest of your life. Think of the menus as building blocks, constructing a good solid program that will last for ever.

As you increase your calorie intake, when you are in maintenance, make the main additions in the form of carbohydrates such as whole grains and cereals, fruit and vegetables; never in wasted 'instant calories' such as sugar. If bread is a special problem for you - as it is for so many over-weight people - count it in. Thin-sliced wholewheat bread was added to the basic minimum diet at the Duke Center, literally by popular demand. Build it into your program, and that's fine. Bread, like wholewheat pasta, rice and potatoes, is a good, nutritious food which leaves you with a feeling of being full. Remember, though, that whilst bread itself is okay, lashings of fat, cream cheese or jelly piled on top are definitely not!

Cholesterol has had a high profile in medical discussions in recent years and everyone now knows that a high level of cholesterol, that fatty, wax-like substance that literally clogs the arteries, contributes to coronary heart disease. There is no need to eliminate cholesterol from your diet completely - very hard to do, in any case - but you do want to limit it. This means keeping an eye on the amount of egg yolk, shrimp and liver you include in your program. Again, this is not a case of 'never again', but of a little of what you fancy - and only occasionally. Structured eating. Planned eating. Portion control. They all lead to success.

You can increase polyunsaturated fats to some extent. Among the fatty acids, these are the 'good guys' which can actually help to lower the amount of harmful cholesterol in the blood. In fact, when the original diet was modified to provide 750 calories instead of 700, the extra 50 calories introduced were in the form of polyunsaturated margarine.

Other concentrated sources of polyunsaturated fatty acids, and therefore the most beneficial form in which to take fat are corn oil, sunflower, safflower and soya oils. It is not recommended that you increase the protein content of the diet. The allowance of 60 grams uses up a high proportion of the calorie total and is adequate. What you can do, of course, is juggle with the way you 'spend' that protein. Since one ounce (roughly 28 grams) of lean red meat is 60 calories, one ounce of poultry is 50 and the same weight of white fish is 35 or even less, you won't need me to tell you that poultry and fish figure prominently in the menu plan, and steak is reserved as a special treat - no more than once a week.

When it comes to branching out and adapting your own favorite recipes to diet-conscious ones, do buy the two essential tools of the trade. First, you'll need a comprehensive book which lists the calorie content of every food, and second, a reliable food scale. You can't control your portions or your calories unless you know exactly what you are planning to put into your mouth. And sorry, folks, but guesswork isn't good enough.

In real budget terms - no pretend budgets, this time - this diet has a lot to offer. The permitted foods, all the grains, vegetables and poultry, are much less expensive than red meats and all the empty-calorie foods, the sweets and snacks. Good news, this! Once you are into the swing of the diet, you will find you have more money to spare. Now's the time to put some aside for a new smaller-size dress or suit, something to look forward to wearing once you've lost that first ten pounds.

Many people comment on the fact that, since this is a low-bulk diet, constipation can be a problem. What we are dealing with here is a change in dietary make-up, and most importantly a change in the amount of food you eat. What happens when you drastically reduce your total food intake is that the body utilizes almost all of it, and at first there isn't a great deal to eliminate. Being the incredible mechanism it is, the body adjusts in about two or three weeks, so don't panic! You may, if you wish, add miller's bran in small amounts, but that's all the added fiber that's allowed. This diet is based on moderation and reason, and strict portion control is essential.

Remember at the beginning of this chapter I stressed the value from all points of view of maintaining a regular three meals a day? Well, I am here to tell you that once you have built that firm foundation -those sound building blocks - you can revert to controlled snacking. In fact, you'll be glad to know that Linda Janick says there is nothing wrong with snacking - as long as you can handle it. Some people, a very few, even do better on snacks - on the principle that they eat little and often. But they do have to be the right kind of snacks. Vegetable sticks, fruit, chicken portions, salads are in. Potato chips, crackers, candy, those great handfuls of peanuts I love so much - they're out.

There's a real psychological problem to snacking that bugs so many people, me included. Somehow the human brain has this ability to overlook what it wants to. And so we snack and then innocently forget all about it. We can even fool ourselves into thinking that all we ate was this wonderful diet meal. And then we wonder why we are not losing weight! I tell you, the human mind is a wonderful thing, but you do have to be there to check up on it. If you know in your heart that you are likely to be fooled - you'll snack and then forget it ever happened - don't do it, ever. The strict three-meal-a-day routine is the one for you.

Forming new habits - and the right ones this time - is what keeping to a new program is all about. Don't make it unnecessarily difficult for yourself. Plan your campaign so that you can win this battle - and the war.

If you eat at home most of the time, structure your kitchen to assist you in your program. Just don't have any foods which are not 'legal' on the shelves or within easy reach.

What about all those illegal foods bursting out of the cupboards today, the day you have made up your mind to start? It depends on your circumstances. Ideally, pack it all up in a box and take it to give to an enemy of yours. You wouldn't give all that stuff to a friend! Take all that canned fruit in syrup, the pâté and canned fish, all that cake in the freezer and say I don't want it in my house any more. 'Happy Christmas! Happy birthday.' Whatever.

If your family eats this kind of thing - and they're all thin - let them eat it when you're not around. But think carefully before you buy the same kinds of food again. Too much sugar, animal fat and salt isn't good for anyone. Growing children need more food than you do, to give them more energy, but they need the right foods.

Use the menus as a rigid guide, and shop for them once a week, or every day, or when it suits you. Make a shopping list and stick to it as firmly as if you hadn't another coin in your purse to spend. Watch your shopping cart very carefully and make sure none of that pâté or other tempting stuff jumps into it.

What about the family while all this is going on? They can enjoy the same foods - and they will enjoy them, I promise you. Give them larger portions, more vegetables and more fruit and let them have extra sweet things if they must. But at least for the first four weeks, ask them to snack while your back is turned. And a word of warning. Never call your new eating program a diet. Tell them what it really is. A gourmet eating experience!

Gourmet is certainly the word. Now more than ever before it matters what your food looks like. Presentation is very important. Food has to satisfy your eyes as well as your stomach, and your eyes are going to look at every meal very critically right now! Make sure every dish passes the eye-appeal test. Dress up main dishes with more herbs, twists of lime and shaped vegetables. Taking extra care about how food looks is very important. It means that you care not only about the food, but about yourself as well. And do you know what the family will say? I'll tell you, from my own experience. 'It's wonderful! You've never taken this trouble with food before. You keep right on with this new gourmet program of yours.'

Your efforts and your enjoyment don't have to stop short after the main course. You will see from the recipe section that you can make fabulous-looking desserts that are perfectly legal. You can make a meringue from sugar substitute that will look just like regular meringue. Fill it with strawberries - nothing wrong with them. It will look beautiful, taste delicious, and no-one will feel deprived. Not even you!

Food really must be fun. Eating just to satisfy real or imaginary hunger is no pleasure. Now you have a more limited selection of ingredients, you have more of a challenge to make them into something fantastic. Rise to it! You have got to look on this new eating experience as something that is fun to do. That way you can take as much pleasure in the anticipation and the preparation as you can in the meal itself. Twice the enjoyment!

Eating in restaurants needs a special campaign, too. I have more to say on that subject in other sections. Here you are up against a number of things. The mood of the occasion, when eating out is often

52

considered some form of luxury or celebration; the food cues all around you - the appetizer table, the dessert trolly going past your table; the 'freebies', the bread rolls, cheese, crackers or relish trays on offer; and the social pressure. Most restaurants have a set meal pattern which is promoted on the menu - drinks, appetizer, soup, salad, entree, dessert, after-dinner drinks - far more than you can normally cope with on your allowance.

If the choice of the restaurant is down to you, go for one where the food is cooked to order. You will find it far easier to handle than a fast-food place or, worse, an all-you-can-eat restaurant. There's always that awful feeling that you should be eating more, to get your money's worth.

Be brave at the outset. Ask the waiter how each dish is prepared. Look around you and see the size of the regular portions. If necessary ask for a half-portion or, a regular thing in the US, ask for a doggie-bag to take the other half home. Ask for all dressings and sauces to be served on the side of the plate, if at all. And if the waiter brings you food you don't want (or at least, that you shouldn't have) smile nicely and ask him to take it away. A pile of golden French fries is too much to test anyone's resolve!

Choose diet soda or other non-calorie drinks. With a spoon of ice and a twist of lime or lemon they look like any other drink. Two large glasses of soda before the meal will help to stop the hunger pangs and make the food a little more resistible.

Strictly speaking there is no reason why you shouldn't structure alcohol into your program, as long as you count the calories and adjust your meals to accommodate it. But here again, at least at the beginning, it is making things harder for yourself. There's nothing like a couple of large martinis to weaken a person's resolve! And then it's oops, who's counting what you decide to eat after that! I found I really had to be confident of my whole program before I could handle a single drink.

If, even without a drink, you really find you're in for trouble when you go to the restaurant, eat a small low-calorie snack just before you go out. Set a calorie limit of around 150 and choose foods from your permitted groups. Half a sandwich can be much more legal than a handful of nuts and nibbles or a chef's special dessert.

Eating out, of course, isn't all soft lights, sweet music and the chef's special. If you go to work every day and are faced with a choice of the 'greasy spoon' up the road, or taking your lunch with you - no problem. Both can be made to fit in with your program. Even a fried chicken meal can be reduced to a reasonable calorie count - you just remove the skin. The good news is that even the hamburger places now are putting in salad bars. With salads, the dressing is always the worst offender, so what you do is order one without dressing or, if you can't face that, take your own low-calorie alternative with you.

Have a word with the waiter or owner if you have a favorite place round the corner, explain what you are trying to do - which is to eat more healthily - and mostly they will be as helpful as possible. After all, what is cooking something to order, with the minimum of oil and no salt, compared to losing a valued regular custumer?

Packed lunches are no problem either. There are so many delicious types of low-fat cottage cheese and low-fat yoghurts all sold in handy cartons; you can have a different one every day for weeks. Just the thing to enjoy with crisp and crunchy vegetable sticks - celery, carrot, cucumber, fennel all keep well in a salad box - and a portion of fruit. Sandwiches can be well within limits - lean poultry, low-fat cheese, variety salads, a handful of dried fruits, they need never be dull.

Many of the recipes are suitable to take in your little brown lunch bag, to eat in the office, in the park, or even in a restaurant or club if you know they serve only the kind of food you can't handle. 'Who would dare?' did you say? I did! And got nothing but praise for my nerve!

I tell you. Once you've made your mind up to lose that weight, and you're pulling for your own success, the whole world is on your side, too. Everyone loves a winner!

Chapter 5

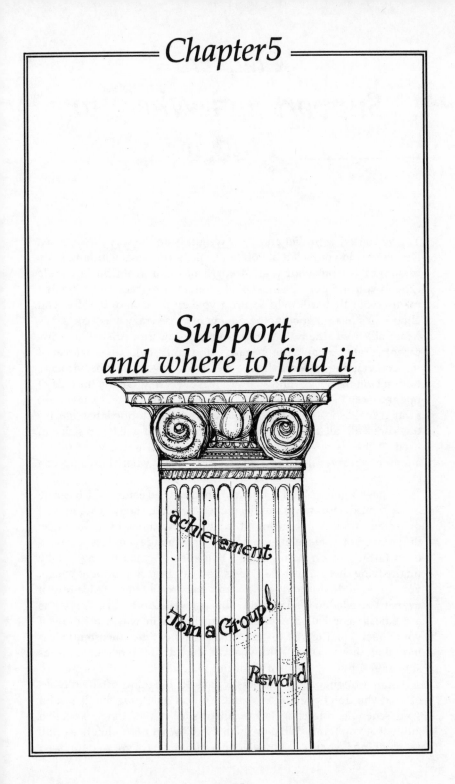

Support
and where to find it

achievement

Join a Group!

Reward

Chapter 5
Support and Where to Find it

You've started your diet and your weight is on the way down, okay. Don't ever kid yourself that you can achieve your goal without plenty of support - from your own strength of mind, from those people around you and perhaps most of all from the program itself. The first main crutch that will help to prop you up is actually the diet you choose. It's just no good going on any of those crazy crash diets. We have all tried them - the eat-nothing-but-fruit diet; the low-carbohydrate regime; the bananas and milk diet, or whatever. I remember going on some strange diet in which you could eat virtually nothing but three eggs and a lettuce leaf every day. On the third day I opened a can of cat food and boy, it smelled good to me! I knew right away I would soon be in big trouble. So I quickly stopped that one. It's the same with all the fad diets. In no time flat you will be so sick and tired of the particular ingredients that you will never want to see another whatever-it-is food again. And that's when bingeing can start.

What is bingeing? Well, it is totally unstructured eating which can be brought on, doctors now think, by the reaction of the body being starved of certain foods for too long. It is also many times brought on by different emotional feelings, rarely if ever by hunger - unless you have been fasting, or on a mono diet. You stick to some boring, totally unsatisfying diet for just as long as you can bear it and then, wham, your mind and your body rebel - and you are clearing the ice-box of every calorie-laden food in sight. This is a well-known fact. There was a medically-controlled experiment in the US in which a group of young men volunteered to eat over a period of time consistently less food than they needed. And what did they do but binge themselves silly after a few weeks. Just went out of control.

Another frequent and less drastic cause of bingeing, often on types of food you don't even like, is guilt. You eat one thing that is not on your schedule, one chocolate eclair or slice of pie, and you feel so guilty that you think, 'What the hell. I've blown it now. I might as well eat anything I want.' I've known of people who have got so depressed at going out of control on their diet that they've come down in the night and eaten a whole chicken with all the trimmings from the fridge, or a large fruit cake by themselves. People who get to this state will eat anything - cold. A feature is that they just never bother to heat it up. They're never going to notice what it tastes like, anyway. Another severe case was the man who ate his daughter's birthday cake piece by piece until there wasn't a bit left and was so ashamed - who wouldn't be - he had to go right out and buy another one before the family found him out. This gigantic craving for food, that has no relation to hunger, is sad. Luckily this doesn't happen to most of us, but it's one of the pitfalls it's as well to know about. Then you can be on your guard and ready to avoid it.

So now we are talking about what's supportive and what's unsupportive. The most supportive thing is what you do right at the outset - make sure that the diet you choose is one which you can live with for the rest of your life. If it's a fad or a fancy diet it's just no good. You won't like it. You won't feel satisfied by it. And sure as anything you won't stick to it.

I know this so well from my own experience, and so I have made a selection of recipes that I feel are utterly realistic to suit all occasions, likes and dislikes. Even people who dislike being on a diet at all! When you come to the recipe section at the end of the book, and all the menus I have chosen for you, you will see that they both look and sound delicious. They look and sound like real food - which is just what they are. Dishes you can serve when you're eating alone, when there's just the family or you are having a company meal. You can have fun in preparing them and pride in serving them. Not only that, you'll find it hard to remember that when food's as good as this you're on a diet at all. Only the scales and the appreciative looks of those around you will remind you that you are.

There's a great deal of argument about whether people on a diet should weigh themselves every day, every week, or less frequently than that. We all know that our inclination is to leap on to the scales every day to check our progress. And that is exactly what I do. I have a really good pair of weighing scales, which I've had checked for accuracy - otherwise there's always the excuse that it isn't me that's gaining weight, it's the scales going out of control again. And I weigh every morning at the same time, when I go into the bathroom. Before I have breakfast. So that the time of day and my weight pattern is constant. For of course it's a known fact that we gain weight gradually all during the day. We are at our lightest in the morning - having fasted all night long - and at our heaviest just before going to bed. So you see it's best for the morale to weigh in the morning, anyway. Then I carefully and honestly write down my weight. So that if I've put on a pound in weight it's there in the book staring me in the face. And I can't ignore it and pretend it didn't happen.

Writing down everything about your weight loss, keeping a personal diary of all these important and intimate details, is tremendously supportive. I honestly don't think I could have achieved what I have without this discipline.

Planning what you are going to eat and then recording it really keeps you on the straight and narrow. Say you are following the menus in this book. Well, you have them there in front of you. You can copy them out, breakfast, lunch and dinner each day, on to cards or into a loose-leaf notebook, and have them with you all the time. At Duke we got a diary specially for this purpose - a piece of forward planning already done for us. At the top of each day's page write the date and your weight.

Once you have this plan for the day, you won't be tempted to buy something that is not on your program. When you're in the grocery store and feeling under great strain in front of the cookie counter, it won't take much of a jolt to remember that a great big box of sweet cookies wasn't on any list you ever wrote out since you started being serious about your weight.

Alongside the foods you are going to allow yourself each day, the fresh fruit, the vegetables, lean meat and poultry, fish, bread and potatoes - funny how people used to think that good wholemeal bread and plain, unbuttered potatoes were villains, isn't it - write down the number of calories. Then you can easily total up your day's intake. At Duke it was about 750 calories a day, but of course you can increase slightly on that if you find you can still lose weight on a higher calorie intake.

Then you need a column for unstructured eating - we called it USE - that's for the tempting foods that you suddenly succumb to in a weak moment. Everybody does it at some time or other, and it's no use thinking you are going to be perfect right from the beginning. The thing is not to feel too badly about it. But to write it down. It's amazing how much less desirable a chocolate ice cream cone seems if you know that for the rest of the day, or the week even, you're going to have to face it in black ink staring up at you from your diary. Suddenly it makes you feel not only guilty but downright uncomfortable. And if you write it all down and then you put on a pound or two in weight, there's no chance you won't know where it came from. Every 250-calorie snack will be there in black and white.

And looking on the bright side, when you lose ten pounds, you're going to know exactly how you achieved it. That will be a tremendous support to you in the future, especially at times when you seem to get stuck at a certain weight, no matter what you do. With the structured and the unstructured food in their separate food columns, the blinkers are off. There's no more being in the dark ever again.

The strange thing is that even in the hardest times I never cheated on the diary. If I was getting really weak - and I did, often, at the beginning - then I would stop keeping the diary altogether. I wouldn't lie to it. I just wouldn't write in it at all for a period. But once I was back on course then everything I ate, every handful of 25 peanuts and every single cookie, went into that USE column. When I saw 250 calories listed down for something I hadn't needed at all - and wouldn't have remembered if it wasn't for the diary - it certainly made me think. Do I really want this extra food so much? Because if I eat it I'm for sure going to write it down. And if I write it down, I'm certainly going to regret it, and feel even more guilty. So maybe I'd best not eat it. Go out and take a walk. Call up a friend for a chat. Anything to take my mind off the temptation. That's how I used to reason myself out of it. The diary certainly helped me to get programmed.

Another way to use a diary as a support system is to make a note of the times and situations when you go 'unstructured' and eat something you shouldn't. If for example you cannot resist the temptation to taste the food while you are cooking - and what self-respecting cook puts food on the table without being sure it tastes good? - limit yourself to one or two small spoonfuls. Tiredness often leads to unwanted snacks. Some people, for example, feel so exhausted when they get in from shopping or work that they really believe they need a snack to perk them up again. Your diary will soon point up the black spots and show you where and when you are going wrong. Then you can plan for it. Have a bowl of raw vegetables ready, reach for them straight away and go on munching celery and carrot sticks until the initial edge of the hunger is gone. Remember that you should always sit down to eat. The rest alone will brush away your original feeling of need.

You might realize for the first time, looking through the entries in your food diary, that a certain person or situation, someone at work or a particular job you loathe doing, always weakens your resolve and ends up in a 250-calorie snack. Oops. Back to those vegetables and diet sodas. The Duke program emphasizes the importance of three meals a day and no snacks, but when stress gets the upper hand, have a legal snack available. You can carry enough around with you in your handbag to cope discreetly and legally with a crisis like this. But without the notes in your diary, the totally honest entries you have made over a period of time, you might never have figured out the cause of these unscheduled trips to the candy store or the fridge.

The theory is that people who are overweight, even if it's only by seven pounds, tend to be unstructured. They find it hard to concentrate on what they eat and why they eat it. Some people really are not very food-aware at all. Now keeping a diary helps you get in the mold of being structured. You write down what you're going to eat for the whole day. And so you really don't have any further choice to make. Once you've made the decision, you don't have to keep on choosing. 'Well, what shall I have for lunch?' Because if you're feeling particularly hungry when you ask yourself that question, and you haven't got a day plan in front of you, you are liable to make entirely the wrong decision. It's like driving through open country without a map. You find it hard to keep a sense of direction and to decide which way to go. But if you've got your day's meals all mapped out, and you know you're going to have this for breakfast, that for lunch and something light and delicious for dinner, then you've got something really good to look forward to. You know it's going to be fun to prepare. You're going to present the dish so that it looks appetizing and attractive. And you know you're going to enjoy eating it, slowly and appreciatively. For me, it's the decision making that's the weakest part of any diet. There are too many paths that lead straight to temptation. Take away the element of choice and I'm on my way!

So the first support step is to find a food plan you know you can stick to - one that is varied and interesting enough to absorb your attention. And the second step is to plan it day by day in advance, and record it in absolute detail as you go through each day. With that extra column for all the wrong turnings you took along the way!

Your diary is the hidden support system that goes on just between you and yourself. But at least at the beginning of your new regime you are also going to need the supportive behavior of those people around you. This can be a problem, because family and friends, thinking they are being helpful, can actually act in a way which is just the opposite. You can't educate each and every one of them into what's helpful and what is not - though you could buy them all a copy of this book! - but you can find out for yourself what behavior is supportive to you. Then, when they do something that makes your task more difficult, just tell them. As I have said, you have to risk being a little blunt with some people if you are to go on succeeding.

Take your immediate family first, for their behavior is going to affect you most. When I used to start on yet another diet, I could see the disbelief in a lot of eyes. If I could have said, 'Heh. I need you to help me believe I can do it. Or at the very least don't roll your eyes to heaven and sigh in disbelief,' I might have achieved my goal sooner. Who knows?

Of course, it's really good for you if those around you recognize that you have changed your eating and activity patterns for the better - and don't try to blow you off course. Though often even your nearest and dearest will try to do this, sometimes for reasons they don't even know about. So here's where you have to understand, and learn to support them in their fears, worries, whatever. Frequently when those close to you see you changing physically and mentally - for now you're losing weight you're beginning to feel good about yourself in a way you haven't done for years - they start to worry. I know of a man who had been married for 20 years to a woman who was very overweight. He was used to this and felt comfortable with the situation. Suddenly she decided to lose weight and she was being very successful at it. The husband soon panicked. She was really going to do it this time. Suppose she wanted sex two or three times a night? That poor man had his own anxieties, and his wife had to give over some time to supporting him!

Losing weight and maintaining your goal isn't always easy, and it is important that your close family and friends realize that, so that they can be on hand to throw you a life-line when you need one. There are all kinds of ways they can show you that they know it - that it isn't an easy row to hoe. Let them praise your efforts as much as they want - who doesn't bask in the glory of praise of any kind. I used to love hearing my husband or my mother boasting to a third party at how successful I'd been - it's like being in third grade and hearing your good examination results being praised to high heaven. You sure feel good about that.

Some of my greatest 'highs' were when I got all dressed up to go to a party and came downstairs and my husband looked at me and went 'Wow!' That sure is supportive. Let them notice the new slim-line you as often as they wish - appreciation of this kind is good for you. But don't let them be constantly asking you how much weight you have lost. This isn't supportive and it can have quite the reverse effect. You can even be made to feel that you are not living up to their expectations of you, and get discouraged to the point of giving up.

When you are on a tight diet regime another thing you can do without is advice from all and sundry. People are all too fond of telling you what you should and shouldn't be eating. If you're anything like me, you've had enough of that in your childhood. Now you're on your diet and in complete control. Let it stay that way.

I've had some bad cases of people close to me acting - without ever realizing it - in a totally non-supportive way. When I was really fat, my husband never said one word about what I ate. He never seemed to notice what food I had on my plate, and certainly never commented. Of course, I was always careful never to let him know the sum total of what I really ate. I was what you call a 'closet eater', although I never went so far as actually eating in a closet! But as most of you will know, we fat people - I'm talking in the past of course - usually do our mainstream eating out of sight of others. That's why those people tend to say to an obese person, 'I don't know why you are overweight. I never see you eat that much.' Of course they didn't see me, I was always very careful about that! In extreme cases, I've known people who didn't even want the girl at the hamburger drive-in to know how much they ate. They'd drive from one to another, buying four or five take-aways each time, eating them in the automobile and driving on to the next. That's when it's really bad.

Anyway, once I had begun to lose weight and it looked as if this time I meant it, my husband John began to take an interest in my food habits. I must say, not too much interest, but just enough to annoy me at times. If I decided I would allow myself a cookie, he just might say, 'What are you doing? You shouldn't eat that!' Or if we were out and I had decided I could handle having one drink without going over the top and having two or three, I would see him watching me and then suddenly out it would come: 'I thought you were supposed to be on a diet!' I figured that I couldn't expect him to know how to handle the situation unless I told him, and got him really on my side in a way which was helpful to me. He got the message, and when I was really being strict with myself at a party he would hand me a glass with soda and a lime and never say a word about it. That's being really supportive.

For years I've had a problem with my step-dad, who has a weight problem himself and should understand. He frequently tries to monitor what I eat. Now here I am, not exactly a child any more, a woman who has finally reduced to a not unreasonable weight. I've done it by myself - which is how we must all do it - and I feel free some-times to eat those foods I usually deny myself. And my step-dad will look at me critically and push food out of my reach down to the other end of the table. I know he thinks he's being helpful, but actually it's just the opposite. For too many years someone else felt the need to control what went into my mouth. And now that I finally have the control I need, people are still trying to wrest it away from me. I need to tell him that his kindly behavior is not only non-supportive, it makes me downright angry. Consider yourself told, Papa!

Something else I found difficult to handle at the beginning was my family and friends snacking in front of me. If you had just given up smoking, people would usually be considerate enough to ask, 'Do you mind?' before lighting up a cigarette in front of you, in case it broke your resolution when it was at a very vulnerable stage. So why don't they give the same consideration to people who have given up candy bars, peanuts, between-meal snacks of all kinds? I used to make my kids eat their candy out of the house, or out of my sight, or at the very least to ask my permission. If I was feeling not too sure of myself that day, I'd say so. Be honest with your friends and family. They obviously do care about you and want to help. But they may not always know how.

The greatest support I had through the whole of my diet adventure was from my daughter Bebe. She seemed to know instinctively what would be supportive and what would be downright destructive to my goal and she encouraged me and bolstered me up whenever I got discouraged. When she was at college she took time to send me cards and letters, and when I came back from a course at Duke she would call me at home to congratulate me over even a one-pound loss. I could be completely open with her when I failed, and we cheered together when I triumphed.

It is important for all of us to realize that there is a great deal of agony, depression and anger as well as the great highs of triumph and success in the weight-loss process. And it's a fact that if we could only let ourselves go more times, let these emotions come out, we would probably be more successful sooner. Bottling up the emotions is a certain recipe for disaster when you're trying to lose weight. You feel angry. You do nothing about it. You just let it ride. But what do you do? You compensate yourself with food. It's the natural comforting thing to turn to. I wish I'd realized this a whole lot earlier. Now if I feel mad at someone's behavior, instead of keeping it all to myself and making straight for the candy jar I say so. 'Heh, that was a pretty rotten thing to say. You sure have hurt my feelings by saying that.' I've got it off my chest. Once I've said it, I no longer feel angry inside, and I don't have any need to compensate myself with food.

Having one confidante who really understands what you are trying to do is the best support anyone going on a diet can have. I was very lucky with Bebe, and she is still my best confidante and friend in the world. A friend who is keeping to a strict eating program at the same time as you is a tremendous support. He or she understands exactly what you are going through because they are going through the same thing. Make it a rule not to ask each other how much weight you have lost. If you want to volunteer the information once a month or so, go ahead. But don't make it a competition. You're not in this to compete. You're in this to do the best you can do. Everyone's body is different and will lose weight at a different pace. If your friend is losing weight faster than you are, it could be very discouraging.

What you can discuss are diet recipes and tricks like using yogurt instead of sour cream. And putting cottage cheese into a blender and whipping it to use for a diet dip. Working out ideas for flavoring cheese dips used to keep me occupied for hours at the beginning. All of these tricks and many more are in the recipe section of this book - but there's still plenty left for you and your dieting friend to work out for yourselves. And I'll bet you will get real fun out of taking your regular recipes and changing them into diet ones. Once you learn the formula you really can make any diet foods that are look-alikes and taste-alikes of family favorites.

I learned fairly early on that when you're looking for this kind of heart-to-heart support it's no use turning to your regular friends. Some of them might be skinny and genuinely not understand what you're on about. Others might have other motives for not helping you along. They might be overweight themselves and jealous of the progress you are making. There are two overweight ladies at my office who have watched me gradually go down and now when I see them they always ask me how my weight's doing. 'Well,' I'll say, 'I guess I'm doing about fine.' And once I said, 'You two are just waiting for me to gain back every bit of my fat, aren't you?' And they laughed and admitted it was so. Seeing me in the office having lost a lot of weight really bothered them. It shows it can be done and now they're feeling guilty about not having tried.

What you really need is one friend who is also on a diet. It's so much easier when you have this kind of support. You know what they say about a problem shared. Well, when that problem's overweight, it sure is a problem halved. Having a friend like this means that you have someone you can always call up if you feel yourself slipping. If you find that you're on the verge of going out of control, and finishing up that cake someone left in the fridge, just call them up. Confess what is going through your mind, food-wise and ask for help. I have to tell you that just talking on the phone, keeping your mind occupied and your hands off that cake for a while, is a help. With luck, by the time you've put the phone down the feeling will have passed.

Don't make the mistake, as so many of us do, of trying to turn your best friend into your diet confidante - not unless he or she has a weight problem too. Your skinny friend will have not the faintest notion of what it means to crave a piece of luscious chocolate cake or pie. This person not only won't understand this compulsive craving, but will now decide they have a looney for a friend! Be careful where you spread your honesty. You want a good big circle of friends left to help you celebrate when you reach your goal!

Eating out at restaurants can burn up quite a lot of your self-support system. But not once you know how to handle the situation. When I was just beginning to feel in control of the situation we went out for a meal to a lovely fish restaurant in Houston. Now as we are only 50 miles from the Gulf Coast, and fish can be a dieter's best friend, I did not anticipate any problems. I certainly didn't anticipate what happened when we got there. Even though we were early we were at the bottom of a long list of diners and had to wait 45 minutes in the bar. That was fine. I had my diet soda with a slice of lime and felt my halo shining brightly. Eventually we got to our table and I ordered a plain grilled fish and a salad with no dressing. Fine. I had coped. I had read the whole menu, enjoyed in my mind a great range of rich dishes, and chosen right within my diet program. And just to be on the safe side, I had brought my own salad dressing with me.

But the chef had other ideas! What actually came up was a huge fried fish absolutely swimming in butter, and a salad with half a cup of standard dressing. Boy, was I hungry by now, and did that food look good! What to do, what to do? 'Eat it, eat it, heaven knows you tried,' my stomach screamed. But my good sense said otherwise. Summoning all the courage I could - and my husband wasn't too pleased at this, I have to tell you - I sent it back. Ten minutes later I was served with what I asked for - and that halo felt even tighter. If I had realized that I might be put in this situation I would never have thought I could handle it. But I did, and came out feeling ten feet tall.

Actually, eating out shouldn't be too much of a problem, especially if you know the restaurant and the type of food they usually serve there. Almost every menu has plain grilled poultry or fish of some kind - if you can only persuade the waiter that that's what you want! A great favorite of mine is an Italian place down the road. When I am dieting seriously - say when I have put back a little weight and need to take it off again quickly - I go there and know I am going to have an absolutely delicious meal with no problems. My 'usual' is red snapper with tomatoes, which is very low in calories. I don't feel the tiniest bit deprived because it tastes so gorgeously Italian!

Another restaurant yarn I must share with you, I think I had rather a novel idea. My sister, Joanna, who was also on a diet, was staying with me when another girl asked us to join her for lunch at the racquet club. Now Joanna and I really could have gone over the top there, and I didn't feel too sure of how to handle it. 'Right,' I said. 'I'm not risking running into any problems there. You and I are going to take our lunch.' And take it we did. I fixed us up two delicious tuna salad sandwiches, all legal, with yoghurt and celery which is just gorgeous, and put them in a brown bag. As we came to the lunch table I saw that our hostess had two other friends there, a doctor and his wife from New York. 'Barbara,' I said, 'this is going to be the cheapest lunch you ever bought me, because we've brought our own. I hope that's all right.' But it was fine with her. She knew I was serious about losing weight, and what a struggle I had had, and she was very supportive. The doctor and his wife were very impressed at our display of mind over matter. And the restaurant sold three good lunches, so they weren't worried. In fact, everybody was happy.

As you would guess, we had a marvelous discussion over that lunch about the whole question of dieting, and that particular doctor was full of understanding. It's a hard thing to say, but I haven't always found that to be the case. When I was faltering at first and looking here, there and everywhere for help and support I naturally thought that after family friends come that other group of people, the professionals. It's a hard thing to say - and of course it does not apply to them all - but there are too many doctors out there in Medical Land who do not have a clue how to approach a fat person concerning weight loss. I have even seen reports of studies that show that some doctors actually dislike their obese patients and tend to ridicule them and drive them away. They just don't want to take the time to understand them and develop proper attitudes for treating these people. It's bad enough that our culture treats obese people like second-rate citizens. But when learned and qualified men and women react badly to what has become a number-one health problem in the country it is ridiculous.

Of course doctors know that obesity leads to severe medical problems. It's too bad that prevention does not have a bigger priority. Or perhaps it is that overweight appears to have such a simple remedy: all you have to do is to eat less. How often have we overweight people heard that one! I have just one straightforward word of advice for you here. Many doctors are understanding and supportive, some are not. If yours is one of those who just don't find your problem interesting enough to catch his attention, get another one!

If you find that it's company and reassurance you're after, you really cannot do better than join one of the weight-loss groups. They fill such a real and human need that wherever you live there is bound to be a group close to your home run by one or other of the large organizations. I found my local group very good at the start, and I certainly lost weight, but found the regular attendance at the classes put too much pressure on me. Perhaps I am a more private person than that, I don't know. But we all react differently. These groups give a very special feeling of belonging to everyone with a weight problem. Fellow members commiserate with you at your disappointments - though the group leader might well have some harsh words to say - and literally cheer at every step you take on the way down to your goal weight. Group discussions are helpful too and can let you know that you are for sure not alone in your problem. There are hundreds and thousands of us out there who have trodden the same path you are treading now!

Whatever the support you get from others around you, you do have to realize right from the outset that your main support is going to come from within yourself. For remember that you are the only person over whom you have complete and absolute control. You can't regulate how others behave towards you, though you can indicate how you would like them to behave. But you can reprogram your mind to think thin and, however difficult it seems at times, to go on thinking thin. The very worst thing you can do, after a round of successful weight loss, is to reward yourself with food. You know the kind of thing. 'I've been so good that I'll just have a slice of angel cake as a reward.' Chances are that after all this deprivation it will taste so good that you'll have another slice, and another. Remember what we said earlier on about bingeing?

Reward yourself in every other way you can. With a new hairstyle. New clothes - and don't wait until you have reached your goal weight. Buy yourself something new in the intermediate size on your way down, even if it means buying cheapo fashions because you know you're soon going to be too *thin* for them. Ladies, it couldn't be easier. Give yourself the luxury of a massage, a facial, have somebody make your face up. You can often get a free make-up in large department stores, so that you will later consider buying their products. Just begin to look at yourself as a beautiful person. When you have achieved some success and lost the first few pounds, you deserve a reward. It used to be more food. Now you know that that's the number-one enemy. But there are plenty of other treats that will all go to make you a more beautiful and confident person. Food never did that, now did it?

Now that I have learned some of these lessons the hard way, my ambition is to help you to get there too. It's the attempt that matters. And never forget, it's a triumph for life when you succeed. I promise!

Chapter6

Fit and Well

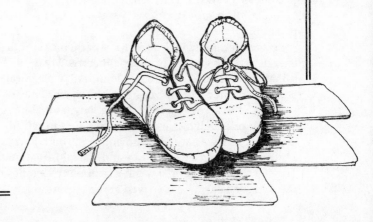

Chapter 6
Fit and Well

Now, don't skip this chapter. It won't hurt, I promise. Though I guess exercise isn't your favorite subject. If it were you'd be reading a book on jogging or, better still, be out there trundling round the block and filling your lungs with fresh air. Don't turn the page in sheer exhaustion at the thought of it until I've had a chance to tell you two things. First, there was no-one in the whole world who hated the very idea of exercise more than I did. And second, if I go for a whole day now without any form of activity I feel really out of sorts with myself and everyone around me. So that must mean something.

My idea of exercise used to be walking from wherever I had parked the car to wherever I was going. And I parked as close to where I was going as possible! When I had lost about 35 pounds (2 stone 7lb) and seemed to be stuck I started hearing about the value of exercise in a weight-loss program. Time was when experts thought you had to walk to kingdom come and back again to lose a single pound in weight. Which gave the lazy ones amongst us all the excuse we needed not to bother. Furthermore, we used to argue, all that running and jumping about did nothing but give us even heartier appetites. We would come in from a good brisk walk feeling full of virtue and make straight for the donuts as a reward. Horrors! Now experts were starting to say that exercise of some kind was essential to any lasting weight-loss program.

So I started looking around for a particular sort of spa - one where exercise was one of the primary concerns. My mother knew someone called Anne Marie Bennstrom who had a place called the Ashram, which translated from the Eastern-Indian word means 'retreat'. I called and talked to a very up-beat young lady, and although I failed to tell her how overweight I was, and she failed to tell me how strenuous their program was, we had immediate rapport. I arranged to arrive on a Sunday in about a week's time and she told me to start walking - now. To my mind a good brisk walk was about two miles in an hour. Boy, was I in for a surprise! I arrived at the airport in L.A. at the appointed time, was picked up along with several other ladies, and whisked up into the Calabasas mountains outside of Los Angeles and the San Fernando valley. My companions all seemed to be frightened and were quite silent. I wondered if they knew something I didn't know! It turns out they did.

When we arrived, each one of us was given a breath test, to see what our lung capacity was, blood pressure and heart-rate tests, and a chat about our general health. Then we were weighed and given what we were told would be our last goodie for a week. Raw vegetables and a delicious dip. You can imagine we all ate accordingly!

After that we were taken on a small three-mile hike to see what sort of shape we were in. It didn't take any three miles for all of us to discern what sort of shape I was in. I was not 'in', I was 'out'. How I ever made that walk and arrived back at the Ashram still alive and in one piece is one of those miracles of pure guts and determination. When I crawled into bed that night I said to myself, 'Mary, whatever makes you think you can survive two days of this, never mind two weeks?' There was no answer.

The girls who looked after us and encouraged us at Ashram, both Swedish, were the most loving, giving, caring people I have ever encountered. They told me later they thought I'd pack up and go home after the first day. But I was determined to do as much as I could, and just a bit more. Maybe I couldn't go on all the same walks with everybody else, but I'd walk every inch as far as I could. And with those girls encouraging me, I stuck with it. When they saw how determined I was, they really pulled out all the stops for me.

In those two weeks, eating an all-raw, no-salt diet, I lost 12 pounds, and, most important of all, I lost 54 inches overall. One day I looked down and saw my feet past my stomach. Was that a high! I left the Ashram having finally faced the fact that exercise has a very important part to play in a weight-loss program. I was definitely 'into' exercise and feeling really fit for pretty well the first time in my life. What more did a girl need to convince her that exercise was the thing? And I found out something else.

Proper exercise, taken regularly, actually cuts the appetite. I did not come in from all that sporting activity ravenous for a huge plate of food. I came in feeling more healthy than I could remember, and with a pleasant interest in food that stopped far short of sheer greed or yearning. So that was another milestone passed and another notch on my way to a new eating pattern.

Since then I have been back to the Ashram five times and each time I was able to do just a little more, until I finally achieved my goal. I went on every walk and made the finishing post in every one. And boy, did I feel good!

Introduction to Duke

This routine set me up well for my first visit to Duke, in Durham, North Carolina. There we were advised that walking was the exercise of choice, a wonderful exercise which, as Dr Nelius pointed out, needs no special training or equipment, and can be done anywhere, at any time. This was no news to me. I had done it, painstakingly and painfully, another place, another time. At Duke we were encouraged to walk at least two miles every day at fifteen minutes each, something which was well within my grasp after what I had been through before.

When Duke first started there was no gym - just as there was no diet kitchen - and no facilities for regular, structured exercise. Then, as research began to show the importance of regular activity, it was gradually introduced to the program, gaining in emphasis all the time.

Since the Center has moved to its new location, things have changed radically and the program is not only more beneficial but a lot more fun. There's now a wonderful pool for daily exercises. Swimming is encouraged in the 'free' time, and there's a coach to teach anyone who can't already swim. The program also includes regular stretching exercises and aerobics - always a popular session. So exercise has now taken its rightful place in the program.

This is in line with the new wave of medical thinking, which shows that diet, or controlled eating, alone is not enough to sustain weight loss. According to recent research, exercise triggers off various changes in the body which actually help it to shed fat. So while you are trotting down to the subway or working out in the gym, encourage yourself with this statistic. Activity increases the rate at which you burn up calories - called your metabolic rate, or the 'tickover rate' - by as much as 30 per cent while you're actually exercizing. And even 24 hours later, long after you've got your proverbial breath back, that rate can still be 10 per cent above normal. And by then you could be sitting down reading the paper!

So what we are finding out is that the effects of exercise are far longer-lasting than were previously imagined. Those of us who hated exercise used to put out all kinds of excuses and anti-activity propaganda, including that old fallacy that 'exercise makes me hungry, so what's the use'! As a matter of fact, that's one of the world's greatest fallacies. Exercise actually cuts the appetite and releases wonderful enzymes which make you feel good physically, as well as emotionally high and morally pure! What more can you ask! I'm telling you, every time I finish my exercise, I can see that halo shining over my head.

As with a weight-loss program, exercise must become a regular part of your daily routine - experts recommend at least thirty minutes a day, four days a week. That amount of exercise will get your heartbeat up to its maximum for your age, and keep it there for a sustained 30-minute period. Thus you will become aerobically fit and give your heart muscle the best possible work out. Just as it's no good going on to a healthy, low-calorie diet for one day and then forgetting all about it, so it's pointless going for a quick run round the park one afternoon and then falling back into your old lazy ways. Only regular exercise has positive benefits. As you get into a regular exercise program, fat cells are squeezed down to their minimum size and muscle tissue grows, which in turn produces more heat than those fat cells ever could, and thus burns up more calories and boosts your all-important meta-bolic rate.

And as with any weight-loss program, your exercise program should be approved by your personal doctor before you begin. A word of caution: Don't start off your exercise program like 'gang busters'. Ease into it gradually until you can sustain it for the approp-riate amount of time and the appropriate weekly periods.

A weight-loss program without exercise presents a very different picture. As every dieter knows, the weight you lose through a low-calorie diet without exercise is in the form of water first, and then fat. Wouldn't you know, fat is the last great flabby thing to be shifted! To get past this obstacle with diet alone you might be tempted to cut down more and more on your calorie intake until you do reach that magical low-weight goal. Don't! This is a terrible mistake and it has been found that a daily intake below 750 calories is harmful, and results in the loss of lean body tissue. In any case, as soon as you start to eat normally the weight will come back again, and this time it will be in the form of fat. Don't I know! I have been on this lose-gain, lose-gain train more times that I can remember. I'd probably still be on it now if I hadn't discovered exercise in time. One of the most important lessons I learned is that once you have reached your goal weight, one of the most vital tools you must continue to use, beside your maintenance program, is regular exercise.

I found this out the hard way. After I had lost 90 pounds, (6 stone 6lb) and maintained that loss for a year I had surgery. I was unable to exercise for almost eight months, and by then I was out of the habit. (A little sideline here - it only takes *two weeks* to get out of shape - isn't that horrible!) I just couldn't get back into exercise for the longest time and sure enough my weight began to creep up. I wasn't eating any more than my maintenance level, but I was gradually putting on weight. Then I got a lot of stress in my life. And a little more weight went on. Thank heaven for the lessons I learned at Duke. Before things got completely out of hand I slipped into the 'relapse' program, gradually started exercizing, and finally went back to regular exercise. And I lost that extra weight. Not only does exercizing keep your weight at that magical level you have chosen for yourself, but it may well lead to a longer and indeed happier life. It's certainly a help in levelling-out stress.

If you have a natural resistance to exercise, you'll have to play tricks on yourself. There are tricks to exercise, just as there are in your weight-loss program. Besides setting up regular exercise periods throughout your week, get into the habit of parking your car in the farthest parking place at the grocery store instead of right next to the entrance. If you drive to work, find a parking lot or space one or two miles from the office, then walk the rest of the way. Instead of always using the elevator to go up one or two floors in your office building, start using the stairs. And after dinner, instead of sitting there watching TV with your partner or whoever, get up from the table and take a walk together. By that time, you won't be so enticed by all the food advertisements you are bound to see as you watch your favorite programs. A study just published shows that children who sit and watch TV for a great many hours are more obese than those who run out and play after school. Even standing on a street corner oggling the girls uses up more calories than sitting in front of the box!

Remember that exercise should be fun - just as your new healthy food should be delicious. You'll never stick to either if they bore you to tears. So if walking briskly round the block or going a stage further and making it a jaunty jog hold about as much delight as eating a piece of damp blotting paper, admit it. Everybody's into exercise these days. There are work-out gyms in pretty well every town. You release a lot of wonderful energy that way, which makes even the toughest routines enjoyable. There are classes you can join for aerobics (exercises that are both continuous and vigorous), tapes and videos with work-out programs you can do at home - to music. If it's rhythm and beat you're after, join an exercise dance group. Swim to music. If you have a strong competitive streak, suppress it as far as your weight loss is concerned - don't try to beat your friends down to a certain goal, just in case you don't make it. That's unnecessarily depressing. But join a local team and play tennis, basketball, whatever you fancy. The standard of your play doesn't matter - every club has a reserves or a third grade. You get just as much exercise running down the side line with the ball whether you eventually score with it or not.

There is no doubt that exercise makes you feel good, not least because of the self-discipline you have taught yourself. In the beginning, when I had to force myself into activity, I felt so very proud and so totally in control of myself. And that, after all, is the key to any life-style change you make. So, grit your teeth and begin. Slowly at first. Remember, you are changing your life and the way you look at yourself, which in turn will change the way you look at the world. And with exercise as part of that life, the world will be a happier and more glorious place to live. And by the way. A lot of stress and pent-up hostility is released during exercise, so your peace of mind will greatly increase as well.

You will even look more beautiful. There's no doubt that exercise is really good for the way you feel. I know that right from the start I *felt* thinner and more beautiful, the very first day. I thought right away, now I've got control of my life and I'm going to look just fantastic. And it happens. Your hair has more sheen to it, your eyes are brighter, your skin has a definite glow. You walk tall, and lighter, as if you're walking on air. As soon as you start exercizing you feel fit. There's a beautiful new you breaking out of that shell. Watch it, fellas!

Chapter 7

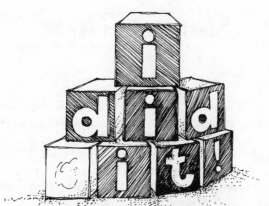

Getting There
and Staying There

Chapter 7
Getting There and Staying There

The way we cope with the setbacks, the plateaus and our whole way of life once we have achieved our weight-loss goal is at least as important as the road we took to achieving that goal in the first place. That is why this is one of the most important chapters in the whole book - it will give you the key to successfully overcoming the pitfalls you are bound to meet - everybody does - at the various points along the way.

It is based on material given me by Ronette L. Kolotkin, PhD, Director of Behavioral Component of the Duke Diet and Fitness Center, and from her superb lecture on Relapse. I found this lecture just about the most significant one I ever heard at the Center. It really struck home with me and many others. Ronnie used to be overweight herself, and is an amazingly caring person; her understanding of the problem knows no bounds. I am deeply grateful to her for her personal kindness and tremendous help.

People like you and me are very hard on ourselves. We tend to be 'either/or' types of people. When we first go on a diet we are convinced we will go all the way. Our enthusiasm is high and we are determined that *this* time, we will stick to it and reach our goal. This kind of enthusiasm is very hard to sustain if you have a lot of weight to lose. One of the biggest things you can do to help yourself is to have a very realistic view of what you are about, and how to cope with the obstacles you will surely encounter. Indeed, just realizing that there *will* be obstacles is the first positive step.

As you notice, the first of these pitfalls is defined as 'relapse'. We use this word rather than 'failure', because relapse is a natural phenomenon which everyone will experience at some time or another. Failure is something you need never know. I will define relapse, and then tell you what failure is. You will see that there is a world of difference.

Relapse is: Gaining weight, having a binge, engaging in unstructured eating, eating a large pizza by yourself, eating out of control for a week or even a month or maybe for just a day or one meal. This is called relapse. *It only becomes failure when you give up.* Sure, you say, that's just semantics. But I guarantee, it's much more than that. It's a way of viewing yourself and reprogramming the old computer to think of yourself as only human and prone to mistakes, just like everybody else.

Failure is: giving up. Failure is saying, 'I'm always going to be a fat person, there's no use trying any more. Failure is burying your head in the sand when the going gets rough and pretending you don't know what you're doing or what you're eating. Failure is no more weighing, no more writing in your diary. It's not looking in the mirror from your neck down. Failure is stopping your weight control classes, avoiding your support system, stopping your exercise program. Failure is waiting until you've gained back all your lost weight plus ten pounds before you do something about it. And most of all, failure is wallowing in feelings of failure and self-pity instead of actively problem-solving your situation.

To be able to stay with a weight-loss program over the long haul, you are going to have to love yourself tremendously. You are going to have to admit that you are human and you will relapse. Maybe once, maybe twice, maybe a lot, a whole lot. But if you were climbing a mountain and you slipped and fell back a little way you wouldn't untie the rope which had helped you make it up this far and say, 'To hell with it. I might just as well fall all the way down.' You would see how far you had come up the mountain and would recognize the steps backward for exactly what they were - a slip.

Redefine success. Success is every single small step you climb up the mountain of weight loss. Success is taking it one day at a time. Success is expecting setbacks and learning how you can best deal with them. Setbacks are a *normal* part of progress. You needn't feel guilty or like a failure after a setback. Coping with setbacks is a real learning experience, not only for losing weight, but for life. Ability to cope with setbacks is the key to long-term success. Remember that a setback is a single independent event which can be avoided in the future. One setback does not a failure make. You must learn to forgive yourself. Because, like the rest of us, you are not a super-person.

So, forgive and forget. Above all, don't feel guilty. Because great big feelings of guilt will require that you punish yourself even further. And you just might decide the punishment is to forget all about the diet and your goal. Chuck the whole thing out of the window and punish yourself with great big helpings of unstructured food. Program this possibility into your personal computer: *Never feel guilty again.* Not about *anything*. Regret, yes. Decide not to do that particular thing again, if possible. But do not feel guilty.

I'd like to say a little more about punishment. When we need comfort we frequently turn to food. Things which perhaps our parents - our mothers mostly - fed us when we needed comfort. 'Fall down and skin your knee? There, there, here's a cookie. That'll make it all better. Love and food are all mixed up. No wonder so many of us are mixed up, too! What you must do is to reprogram your old computer now. Food must no longer be a comfort or substitute for love. Food which is not on your program must now become the enemy. It *is* the enemy to all your golden plans.

If you are disappointed in love, your job, your kids, no longer turn to food. That would be punishing yourself, not the cause of your disappointment. Think of unstructured food as something that does bad things to you - it does, it makes you fat - and try to put it in the rightful place in your life.

If, however hard you try to tell yourself these things, you do go off the rails - and you will - just start again. It's like taking a clean sheet of paper. You just turn it over and start afresh. You say, 'Today is the first day of the rest of my life.' It's just not worth giving up all the effort you have made so far. By now you might have lost five or six pounds. And so you get on the scale the next morning and you may have gained three pounds. Crisis! But turn this catastrophe into a real help.

For instance, the next time you go to a dinner party, try to remember how you felt when you got on the scale. Maybe that will deter you from eating more than you've planned. Keep telling yourself that however delicious the food in front of you may be, it just isn't worth the large bout of depression you'll surely get if you eat too much of it. It really isn't. Not if your main priority is to lose weight rather than see how much you can eat, and how often!

I remember going out of control in a completely unexpected way once. I went into a discount store and there in the middle of the aisle was a huge display of candy bars - five for a dollar! Now is that a bargain or is that not a bargain? So I thought, well I'll buy some of those for my housekeeper's children. So I brought them home and of course who was the first child to get them? That's right, me! And not only one. I ate one, two, three, just as if I didn't know what I was doing. Suddenly, it hit me. What was I doing? I came to my senses and shoved the remaining candy bars back in the sack and gave them to my housekeeper, fast. And to think her children had been my excuse for buying them! Of course, what had really happened was that faced with the combination of candy and a bargain, I just couldn't resist. I love a bargain nearly as much as I love candy!

How many times have mothers bought donuts and all kinds of stuff for the kids, and when the children get home from school there's nothing left? We've all done it. It's so easy to fool yourself. And it gives you twice as many reasons for feeling guilty. One, you have sort of gone out of your mind, just when you thought you were getting to be so strong. Two, you've deprived the kids of something that was rightfully theirs - because never forget that's who you bought the things for in the first place. Just don't feel guilty and come down hard on yourself. Think it through. Understand why you did it. Look long and hard at how you feel about turning off your mind like that. You're not feeling too good about it, obviously. Remember those bad feelings so that next time you see a *bargain* you will recognize it for what it really is: an excuse to go off your program. Is any candy bar or cake worth that? None that I've ever met!

Sometimes certain foods really haunt you as you're on your way down to your goal weight. If you're extremely lucky your dream food will have a low-calorie and almost legal substitute. Take baked potatoes split in half and oozing with butter. That used to be one of my particular favorites. Well, you can have the potato, that's perfectly legal. It's a good and nutritious food. In fact, it's got to be the finest thing you can eat as far as filling you up is concerned. But instead of all those melting calories, fill it with cottage cheese or yoghurt and vegetables like broccoli, carrots and mushrooms. It's just about the same thing. And you've stayed structured.

Some things do not have such easy substitutions. Chocolate eclairs, for instance. Isn't it awful how many overweight people have this really deep-down craving for chocolate this and chocolate that? I wouldn't mind betting that chocolate alone is guilty for the continuing problems of a vast majority of people. Chocolate cake. Chocolate pudding. Chocolate ice cream. Candy bars. I have often heard people say that if they thought they could never have a piece of chocolate cake again, they'd never start a weight-loss program in the first place. Chocolate means that much to them.

Once you have had a few relapses, and have found out that you can handle them with great success, it's okay to give in to those cravings. But give in to them in a structured way. Plan that chocolate eclair which has been on your mind for over a month. You have now made a choice to have it. You therefore have control over yourself. There's all the difference in the world between planning and structuring a food not known to be in your regular plan, and coming upon a bakery, turning off your mind and watching yourself eating unstructured foods as if you couldn't help it.

Walk into the bakery, and smell all those smells which you have been denying yourself for so long. Take a long time to pick and choose exactly what you are going to have to satisfy this month-long desire. Savor every small happening concerned with this pastry. I'll bet you money that it will be one of the greatest experiences of your life. For one thing, it is a real special happening. You haven't had anything like this in a very long time. If you were eating pastries by the handful every day and feeling guilty and depressed about it, it wouldn't be a pleasure, it would be a real downer. But now, maybe for the very first time in your life, you are guilt free. You are in total charge of what you are doing. You have made a conscious choice and because it is something you have not had in a long time it will taste like no other pastry you have ever eaten.

Take your time eating it. Savor every bite. It may be a tiny relapse, but in reality it is structured/unstructured eating done by plan, done by choice, and enjoyed immensely. Once it is over with, remember the experience not with depression, but with pride. You have met the enemy, and made him a friend.

I would like to stress here that many people on a weight-loss program have an inordinate fear of seeing, smelling or reading about certain foods which they crave. They are afraid they will have one glimpse, sniff or bite, or hear one word and go completely out of control. I used to fantasize that I would wake up one morning and be back where I started if I ate one morsel which I did not plan. Even I know it's impossible to gain 90 pounds overnight! But, there you are. It's irrational, but it happens. If that kind of thing happens to you it could be worthwhile structuring in a heretofore forbidden treat, just so that you can see that you *can* handle it. Take a friend with you into the bakery or wherever if you need support. You need to learn how to conquer these fears, and how to eat these foods in a controlled way, otherwise they will eventually lead to your downfall. Remember, this is a plan for life and along the way of your weight-loss adventure you will be learning many things which can help you cope with life in general.

Coping Strategies

Ronnie says your goal is life-style change and long-term habit change, rather than a temporary, short-term reduction in food intake. There is no magic - controlling your weight requires effort, active problem-solving and making choices. Too many over-weight people look upon weight-control as a moral issue. No scarlet woman could feel more shame, no bank embezzler more full of guilt than the dieter who has slipped off his planned weight-loss program.

It is *not* a moral issue, folks. So look at your human failings for what they are. Instead of saying. 'I cheated,' say 'I overate'. Rather than, 'I was bad. I am a bad person,' say, 'I ate cheesecake this week, as planned, and I loved it.' I know from personal experience that even when I structure in a treat, a tiny little voice, even now, accuses me of being greedy and doing something wrong. It's a hard issue to come to grips with because it is one of the behaviors we learn. And so we have to work very hard on understanding what we are saying to ourselves and change it as quickly as we can.

These bad person, bad week-type phrases are destructive conversations, and must be brought out into the open and done away with. Instead of saying, 'Is butter legal?' say, 'I need to make a decision about whether or not I want to spread butter on my toast.' All these strategies put *you* and not circumstances in control of your weight-loss program. Rather than saying, 'I blew it,' say, 'I had a high-calorie week.'

Progress is often slow and irregular, Ronnie assures us. 'Progress involves setbacks. Progress is defined by looking at the date, not at your feelings. Progress involves more than just weight loss.'

It is very important to realize that your goal is not to develop self-control so much as to succeed. Instead, learn to control your environment rather than being controlled by it. If pastries and cakes drive you crazy, don't go into a bakery unless you have it planned and written in your diary. If you can't resist chocolate, don't volunteer to make the fudge and brownies for the church bake sale. Whether you know it consciously or not, a little voice inside is saying, 'Well, I'll be able to have a taste and no-one will see me.' If no-one sees you, does that mean you didn't do it? You can't fool yourself with that old trick any more.

If you are going to drink a diet soda, have it already in your house. Don't stop by the store on your way home to buy it for a certain occasion. Who knows what else you're going to buy while you are there? It is most important to 'fat proof' your house by eliminating high-calorie foods; get rid of foods that you regularly overeat; see that you have a stock of low-calorie food and drink readily available to you and, very important, ask family members to be responsible for their own high-calorie snacks and treats. If they really need them, that is.

Get your shopping habits into line with your new program. Buy only what you plan to eat. If you have structured in an ice-cream cone for yourself, go to the ice-cream parlor and buy only the one cone - unless other family and friends are around, of course. Don't go to the donut shop for 'coffee'. Why torture yourself this way? Are you really into pain? Above all, don't think it's silly and childish not to have enough control over eating sweets or nuts that are in the house. Just don't have them there. You have this problem now because you thought you could cope with these things, and most of the time you found the temptation was too great. This plan-ahead strategy is smart because it works. Remember, your goal is to succeed, not to develop super-human powers of control!

One of the best coping strategies is learning to anticipate vulnerable times. The earlier you are aware that you are involved in a chain of events which make you vulnerable to eating out of control, the sooner you can intervene. Identify those occasions when you will probably have a hard time controling your food. Do you over-eat when you're tired? Most of us tend to do that. Do you go out of control, as so many of us do, when under pressure? Many times when people are physically run-down or sick they are prone to make up for it by over-eating or, just as bad, eating the wrong foods. Stress and family conflicts are frequently associated with over-eating. Remember, when you over-eat because you are mad at someone, the 'madder' never gains any weight. It's always the 'maddee'. I believe I've just invented two new words!

Another 'whoops, here comes trouble' situation that needs facing fair and square is when you have a wedding reception or a business party coming up with an 'all you can eat' buffet. Practise your coping strategy in advance. Close your eyes and envisage all that fantastic food, and find the salads, the cold shrimp, the roast beef, the vegetables, all of which you can eat, in suitable amounts. See yourself approaching the table and getting a small plate, not a dinner plate. Write in your diary exactly what you are going to have. Even though you don't know the precise menu, most buffets have roughly the same type of things. In other words, it's the same planning which a general would do before going into battle. He doesn't know the exact location or strength of the enemy army, but he has a good idea, and so is able to make his plans for victory. Planning before the event is one of the best coping strategies you can employ.

Taking your mind off food and on to other things entirely is another helpful coping strategy. Ronnie describes it as 'engage in positive self-indulgence with non-food items'. Do a lot of things you want to do, and try and cut down on the amount of 'shoulds' in any one day. Indulge in an orgy of television if that's your thing. Call up a friend and plan a non-food outing to the movies or a game. Disconnect food from activity in your mind. Redirect your thinking away from food and on to all the other pleasures in life. Count your non-food blessings. There are plenty of them!

One of the most important things to say here is, do not let the scale rule your feelings of well-being. 'I feel good today, because I lost a pound,' and 'I feel rotten today because I didn't lose an ounce, or I gained,' are positively unhelpful reactions to your regular weigh-in. A lot of people find this one of the hardest behaviors to change. They're so geared to weight-loss that it becomes the be-all and end-all. Remember, losing weight is only a part of this program. You are also going to change the way you handle food, think about yourself and cope not only with weight-loss, but with life itself.

Changes in thinking habits often precede changes in eating habits and weight loss. 'Thinking habits, eating habits and exercise habits go hand in hand,' Ronnie tells us. People are as different from each other as, well, as there are numbers of people. Your next-door neighbor will not lose weight in the same way that you do. You are unique in many ways, and this is only one of them. Don't compare yourself with anyone else. Cherish your own uniqueness, and don't moan and groan because Martha loses faster than you do. Tailor your eating habits to suit your own life-style. For instance, if you need to eat your main meal at lunch rather than dinner, do so. The same principle applies to your physical activity. Take up whatever exercise gives you most pleasure and, equally important, the one you are most likely to stick with, whether it be walking, or aerobics, or swimming. This is finding pleasure in things other than food, and very beneficial things at that.

If in spite of trying your hardest, you realize you have coped unsuccessfully, there is no need to hate yourself and give up. You are not a failure. You have simply coped unsuccessfully with a very difficult situation. Let's face it, we all cope unsuccessfully with many difficult situations in life. Forgive yourself and go on. Start self-monitoring and planning immediately after the setback. *Don't wait until Monday.*

First of all, list previous successes. If you want to have it in black and white, make a list of every time you *did* cope well, and write it down so that you can read it now. Examine the sequence of events which led to the setback and rehearse alternative coping strategies for the future. Learn from your setback. Seek support from friends and, if need be, professional people. While passive yielding to the situation is easier than active coping, only active coping can bring you long-term success. No more waiting for magic. No more wallowing in self-pity and feelings of approaching failure. Make active choices rather than excuses.

Getting Stuck on a Plateau

However rigidly you stick to your daily calorie intake for weight-loss and avoid all the pitfalls, there is bound to come a time when, for some reason or other, your weight reaches a plateau. Now I've known people who don't go on plateaus. And I've known people who have experienced them more than once. It is a very depressing thing to have to go through. Especially when you know you are doing the *right thing*. Sometimes your weight will even go up - God forbid - when you've been utterly structured; something which so many of us do experience, that it is as well to be prepared in your mind. This can be due to a number of causes related to the fact that the human body operates on a regular cycle, and our bodies are more likely to retain fluids at some times than others.

So, you've been doing everything exactly right, you step on the scale and - oh no - you've put on two pounds. You haven't gone out of control. Has all your effort been for nought, and on and on! Cool down there! Stop being an all or nothing person. Almost everybody who goes on a regular weight-loss program encounters this weight plateau or gain at some time or another. At the beginning, when the body is shedding excess fluids fairly rapidly, weight goes down at a very satisfying rate. After that progress usually slows down to an average of about two or two-and-a-half pounds a week. Some lose more, some less. Everybody is different. Then, when everything seems to be going fine, you hit this plateau. It is a perfectly natural thing and can be simply explained.

Your body is simply adjusting itself to what has happened so far. If you have only a small amount of weight to lose - say ten pounds - this plateau may never happen. But if you have 20 or 30 pounds to lose, it may well happen. At these times the body is sort of pausing and taking stock of what is going on. It's holding on to fluid and even to fat. It will decide when to start letting go again. Your job is simply to keep on with your program. If it depresses you too much, don't weigh every day. Wait a couple of days and see what has happened. Plateaus can last as long as ten days or be as short as two days. The important thing for you is to be prepared and deal with the situation constructively. If the plateau goes on for as much as ten days, add 50 or even 100 calories to your breakfast or lunch. It's a way of fooling your body into starting the weight-loss again. Keep those calories in your program if you continue to lose. The important thing to remember is: Keep on with your program, try not to be depressed, and don't use the plateau as an excuse to go off the program.

Maintainance

Reaching your goal weight is like reaching another plateau - the one you will stay at for the rest of life. So this one is welcome. What this goal weight is will depend to a large extent on what image you have of your own body. And, as we have seen, this depends on a number of factors: how you viewed yourself as a child, your upbringing and even fickle things, such as your mood on any particular day. Or, of course, your doctor may have given you a goal weight for your health's sake.

Maintaining this magic weight once you have reached it takes the same kind of perseverance and determination that it took you to get there in the first place. This is where so many 'diets' fail. Now you have the weight off, what do you do? The Duke Diet has this carefully planned and programmed. That's why we call it a plan for life. A diet has the connotation of something which, once you've lost the weight, you are finished with, and can 'go off'. The Duke Diet goes on helping you and supporting you.

Once you have reached your goal weight, continue to weigh every day and watch what you put in your mouth as before. Begin to add 100 calories at a time to your program. Add more of the foods you are already eating. Increase your portions, but never by guess or by golly! Weigh your food as you have before.

The foods you add must be nutritious, healthy, tasty foods - exactly the kind you have been eating, only more of them. After you have raised your calories to your goal weight in pounds x10, you should be maintaining your goal weight. Continue to structure your food - it should be second nature to you now. And now you can begin to structure in some of those foods which you have not allowed yourself all the time you were on a weight-loss program. Once a week, twice a week, but the key is structure. Never, never again eat unconsciously. That is the road to rack and ruin. You must be ever alert to what you are putting into your mouth. If you let unawareness creep into your eating plans ever again you are in for big trouble.

Imprint this on your mind: Once you have reached your goal weight, don't reward yourself with ever-increasing amounts of unstructured foods. That's how you got this shape in the first place!

There's one vital thing which won't be too much help at this stage: you are likely to get much less support from those around you. While you were on the way down, people were more aware of what you were trying to achieve and - hopefully - some of them were very supportive. Now that you have stunned them all by your success and the new-look you, family and friends are likely to switch their attention away from you. Quite likely they will stop complimenting you about how nice you look. After all, it isn't news any more. And in all probability, if they think about it at all, they will feel you can cope on your own now.

What you have to remember is that your goal weight is not the end. It is only the beginning of the second part of your program. And the second part of the program will set the pattern for the way you will eat for the rest of your life. If you're not too sure about that, remember what I said earlier. That the Duke Diet is 'A Plan for Life'. And that's just what this book is giving you.

This chapter could well have been called 'slipping backwards, getting stuck and staying where you want to be'. The Duke Diet has strategies to cope successfully with all those situations.

From day one when you start your weight-loss program, through the 'high' you experience when at last you achieve your goal weight, and then on through that permanent plateau called maintainance, don't forget to love yourself. Praise yourself. And forgive yourself. Like the rest of us, you are only human. And don't forget that a lot of us have been down that path before, and are out here pulling for your success.

Chapter 8

Calorie-wise Gourmet Meals

Introduction

Diets work only if they are delicious - and varied. I have learned that the hard way, trying to stick with monotonous regimes that have had me screaming, and rushing for the cream cake, in a matter of days.

This one is different. I have gathered the recipes from the Duke Diet and Fitness Center, and from my own highly experimental kitchen. And I have counted the calories, and arranged the dishes for you in an easy-to-follow menu form.

That way, you have a complete menu plan - from breakfast each day through to supper - for a whole month. No tantalizing decisions to make. No dreary sums to do. Just the delight of anticipation, and the joy of sharing these tempting meals with friends and family. Whether they need to lose weight or not, they will give you full marks for your irresistible gourmet meals.

Glossary

This 'dictionary' of American and British cookery terms may be helpful to readers on the other side of the Atlantic.

AMERICAN	BRITISH
baking apple	cooking apple
baking pan	baking tin
broil(er)	grill
catsup, diet	if unavailable, use tomato purée
cheesecloth	muslin
eggplant	aubergine
green onion, or scallion	spring onion
ground	minced
ground round	minced round beefsteak
non-stick spray	a lecithin-based aerosol spray to use in place of a non-stick pan. If you cannot obtain the spray, and have no suitable non-stick pan, very lightly brush a conventional pan with oil, or line baking pans with non-stick silicone paper.
oatmeal	porridge oats
paper towel	kitchen paper
part-skim milk	semi-skimmed milk
plastic wrap	cling film
skillet	frying pan
squash	any kind of gourd-like vegetable - for example zucchini (courgette)
tomato paste	concentrated tomato purée
wax paper	use greaseproof or non-stick silicone paper
zucchini	courgette

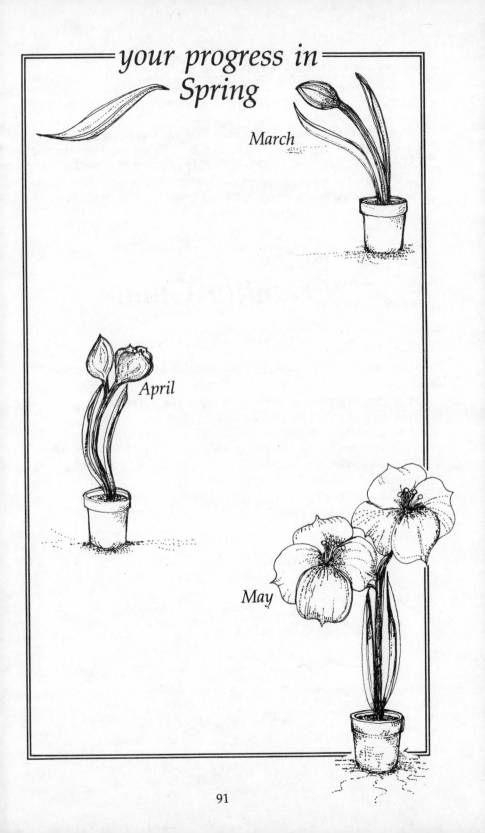

your progress in
Spring

March

April

May

91

Cook's Notes

Throughout the recipes in the book, the measurements are given in three columns: American (US) measures in the left-hand column, and Metric and Imperial measures on the right of each ingredient. Use only one column of measures when making each recipe. The conversions are as accurate as possible, but not exact, and problems would arise in switching from one column to another.

Quantity Guide

1 serving of each recipe (unless otherwise stated) is one-quarter of the whole
1 serving of green vegetables is ½ cup/100 g/4 oz
1 serving of potato is half a 125 g/5 oz potato
1 serving of fruit is half a small banana, medium apple, pear, peach, orange or grapefruit, or ½ cup/100 g/4 oz mixed fruits such as fresh strawberries, raspberries, grapes and so on, or ½ cup/100 g/4 oz canned fruits in unsweetened juice
1 serving of rice is ½ cup/100 g/4 oz cooked weight.

SOUPS

Quick Vegetable Soup

Serves 4

*25 calories
per serving*

1 cup	*tomato juice, unsalted*	225 ml	8 fl oz
⅓ cup	*water or unsalted stock*	75 ml	5 tbls
½ cup	*button mushrooms, sliced*	25 g	1 oz
⅓ cup	*celery, chopped*	50 g	2 oz
⅓ cup	*carrot, sliced*	50 g	2 oz
3 tbls	*green pepper, seeded, cored, chopped*	3 tbls	3 tbls
¼ tsp	*dried oregano or basil*	¼ tsp	¼ tsp
1 pinch	*garlic powder*	1 pinch	1 pinch
1 pinch	*black pepper*	1 pinch	1 pinch
	few strips thinly pared lemon peel (optional)		

Put all the ingredients into a saucepan. Bring to the boil, cover the pan, lower the heat and simmer gently for 15 minutes, or until the vegetables are tender.

* In place of the vegetables listed above, you may substitute a similar amount of any low-calorie vegetables.

Creamed Consommé

Serves 4

*75 calories
per serving*

2 cups	*condensed canned consommé*	475 ml	16 fl oz
2 cups	*buttermilk*	475 ml	16 fl oz
1 tbls	*fresh parsley or chives, chopped*	1 tbls	1 tbls

Heat the consommé just until warm, then stir in the buttermilk. Refrigerate until cold. Sprinkle each serving with parsley or chives.

Chicken Soup

Serves 4

*110 calories
per serving*

4 cups	water	950 ml	1½ pt
½	small chicken, skinned	½	½
1	medium potato, peeled and quartered	1	1
2	small carrots, halved	2	2
¼ cup	fresh parsley, chopped	4 tbls	4 tbls
¼ tsp	salt	¼ tsp	¼ tsp
	black pepper to taste		
4	celery sticks, halved	4	4

Put water and chicken into a large pan, bring to the boil and simmer for 30 minutes. Add vegetables and seasoning and continue to simmer until vegetables are tender. Remove chicken and set aside to cool. Blend the vegetables and stock and return the purée to the pan. Remove chicken from bone, dice and stir into the vegetable purée gently. Taste the soup and adjust the seasoning if necessary.

Gazpacho

Serves 4

*75 calories
per serving*

1 lb	canned tomatoes, unsalted	450 g	1 lb
1 cup	cucumber, peeled and chopped	150 g	5 oz
¾ cup	green pepper, chopped	150 g	5 oz
¼ cup	onion, chopped	40 g	1½ oz
2 cups	Bloody Mary mix	475 ml	16 fl oz

Coarsely mix the tomatoes, cucumber, green pepper and onion in a blender, making sure that the vegetables do not turn to a purée. Turn into a large serving bowl or soup tureen and stir in the Bloody Mary mix. Refrigerate and serve cold.

Senegalese Soup

Serves 4

65 calories
per serving

1 tbls	margarine	15 g	½ oz
1 tsp	curry powder	1 tsp	1 tsp
1 tbls	flour	1 tbls	1 tbls
1½ cups	unsalted chicken stock	350 ml	12 fl oz
1 tsp	paprika	1 tsp	1 tsp
¼ cup	skim milk	4 tbls	4 tbls
1 tsp	fresh chives, chopped	1 tsp	1 tsp

Melt the margarine in a saucepan and stir in the curry powder and flour. Cook for about 1 minute, then slowly add the stock. Bring to the boil, stirring. Remove from the heat and when the boiling has subsided, add the paprika and milk. Return to a very low heat and cook for a few minutes, stirring constantly and not allowing the soup to boil. Refrigerate until cold. Sprinkle each serving with chives.

Vegetable Beef Soup

Serves 4

55 calories
per serving

2½ cups	water	600 ml	1 pt
2 oz	lean stewing beef, diced	50 g	2 oz
¾ cup	potatoes, peeled and diced	125 g	4½ oz
¼ cup	parsnip, diced	25 g	1 oz
½ cup	green beans, trimmed	25 g	1 oz
½ cup	canned tomatoes, unsalted, chopped	125 g	4 oz
½ cup	tomato juice, unsalted	125 ml	4 fl oz
	herbs and seasonings of choice to taste		

Put the water and meat into a large pan. Bring to the boil, reduce the heat and simmer for 1 hour, skimming off any scum as necessary. Add the remaining ingredients and continue simmering for a further 1 hour.

* For a thick hearty version of this, purée the soup in a blender until fairly smooth, then reheat to piping hot before serving.

Spinach Soup

Serves 4

40 calories per serving

½ tbls	butter or margarine	7 g	¼ oz
1¼ cups	onions, chopped	175 g	6 oz
½ lb	fresh spinach	225 g	½ lb
2 cups	unsalted chicken stock	475 ml	16 fl oz
2 tbls	fresh parsley, chopped	2 tbls	2 tbls
½ tsp	salt	½ tsp	½ tsp
⅛ tsp	ground cinnamon	⅛ tsp	⅛ tsp

Melt the butter in a non-stick pan. Add the onions and cook gently for about 7 minutes until light brown. Meanwhile, wash the spinach thoroughly, then drain and cook it, covered, until limp. (No need to add water, just use what clings to the leaves.) Put the onion and spinach into a blender and work to a purée. Turn the purée into the pan and add the stock, parsley, salt and cinnamon. Simmer gently for 10 minutes. Serve hot or refrigerate and serve cold.

* Serve the chilled soup with 1 tbls plain low-fat yoghurt swirled on the top, and sprinkle with paprika. Add 20 calories per serving.

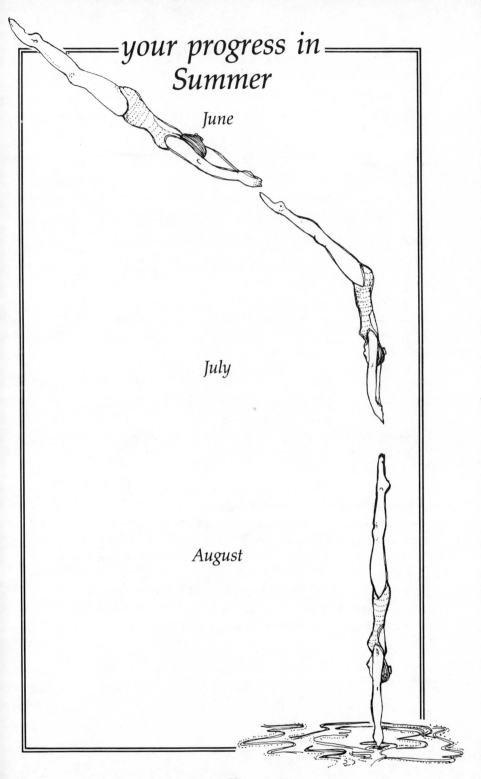

June

July

August

SALADS

Gazpacho Mold

Serves 20-40

15-30 calories
per serving

1 envelope	*unflavored gelatin*	1 envl	1 envl
1½ cups	*tomato juice (unsalted)*	350 ml	12 fl oz
1 tbls	*vinegar*	1 tbls	1 tbls
1 tsp	*paprika*	1 tsp	1 tsp
½ tsp	*dried oregano*	½ tsp	½ tsp
¼ tsp	*ground cumin*	¼ tsp	¼ tsp
⅛ tsp	*Tabasco pepper sauce*	⅛ tsp	⅛ tsp
1	*garlic clove, finely chopped*	1	1
1½ cups	*fresh tomatoes, finely chopped*	250 g	9 oz
½ cup	*cucumber, finely chopped*	65 g	2½ oz
½ cup	*green pepper, finely chopped*	125 g	4 oz
½ cup	*celery, finely chopped*	65 g	2½ oz
2 tbls	*onion, finely chopped*	2 tbls	2 tbls

In a small bowl sprinkle the gelatin over ½ cup/125 ml/4 fl oz of the tomato juice and let it soften for about 5 minutes. Stand the bowl in a pan of water over low heat and stir for about 3 minutes until the gelatin has dissolved. Slowly add to the remaining juice, stirring constantly. Add the vinegar, spices and Tabasco. Refrigerate until partially set (about 1 hour), then fold in the garlic and chopped vegetables. Turn into a mold or individual molds and refrigerate until set, about 4 hours.

Cranberry Celery Mold

Serves 4

about 30 calories per serving

1 tbls	*powdered gelatin*	1 tbls	1 tbls
½ cup	*cold water*	125 ml	4 fl oz
1 cup	*apple juice*	225 ml	8 fl oz
1 tbls	*lemon juice*	1 tbls	1 tbls
⅔ cup	*cranberries, coarsely chopped*	125 g	4 oz
⅔ cup	*celery, chopped*	75 g	3 oz
	lettuce leaves to garnish		

In a small bowl, sprinkle the gelatin over the water and let it soften for 5 minutes. Stand the bowl in a pan of water over low heat and stir for about 3 minutes until the gelatin has dissolved. Slowly pour the gelatin into the apple juice, stirring to blend well. Refrigerate until almost set. Add the lemon juice, cranberries and celery. Spoon into a serving mold (or 4 individual molds) and refrigerate until set. Arrange lettuce leaves on a serving plate and unmold the gelatin on top.

Carrot, Pineapple and Raisin Salad

Serves 4

100 calories per serving

2 cups	*carrots, grated*	250 g	9 oz
1 cup	*crushed pineapple canned in juice*	275 g	10 oz
¼ cup	*seedless raisins*	40 g	1½ oz
½ cup	*unsweetened lemon yoghurt*	125 g	4 oz

Put the carrots, pineapple and raisins into a bowl. Add the yoghurt and toss gently to mix. Cover and refrigerate for at least 3 hours before serving, to combine the flavors.

Bean Salad

Serves 4

25 calories
per serving

1 cup	canned wax beans, drained and sliced	150 g	5 oz
1 cup	canned green beans, drained and sliced	150 g	5 oz
¼ cup	onion, chopped	40g	1½ oz
¼ cup	cider vinegar	4 tbls	4 tbls
⅛ tsp	black pepper	⅛ tsp	⅛ tsp

Toss the beans and onion with the vinegar and black pepper. Cover and refrigerate for at least 3 hours before serving.

* Use fresh beans when they're in season, cooking them lightly to keep the color and crunchiness.

Cottage Cheese Surprise

Serves 4

180 calories
per serving

2 cups	low-fat cottage cheese	450 g	1 lb
	sugar substitute equivalent to 1 tsp sugar		
1	apple, cored and diced	1	1
1	small banana, thinly sliced	1	1
1 cup	sliced peaches canned, drained	225 g	8 oz
1 tsp	sunflower seeds	1 tsp	1 tsp

Mix the cottage cheese and sugar substitute together. Combine all the fruit with the cottage cheese, sprinkle with the sunflower seeds and serve at once.

Potato Salad

8 oz	*new potatoes*	225 g	8 oz
3 tbls	*low-calorie mayonnaise*	3 tbls	3 tbls
4 tsp	*skim milk*	4 tsp	4 tsp
2 tsp	*lemon juice*	2 tsp	2 tsp
2 tsp	*cider vinegar*	2 tsp	2 tsp
¼ tsp	*thyme*	¼ tsp	¼ tsp
1 pinch	*garlic powder*	1 pinch	1 pinch
1 pinch	*black pepper*	1 pinch	1 pinch
2	*small hard-boiled eggs, whites only,*	2	2
	chopped		
3 tbls	*celery, chopped*	3 tbls	3 tbls
3 tbls	*green pepper, chopped*	3 tbls	3 tbls
3 tbls	*onion, chopped*	3 tbls	3 tbls
3 tbls	*button mushrooms, chopped*	3 tbls	3 tbls
2 tsp	*fresh parsley*	2 tsp	2 tsp

Cook the potatoes just until tender. Drain, and when cool enough to handle peel them, if desired, and dice. While the potatoes are cooling, blend the mayonnaise with the milk, lemon juice, vinegar, thyme, garlic powder and pepper. Pour the dressing over the warm potatoes and add the egg whites, chopped vegetables and parsley. Gently toss until all the pieces are coated. Cover and refrigerate for at least 4 hours before serving.

Marinated Vegetable Medley

Serves 4

*25 calories
per serving*

1 cup	*cauliflower florets*	125 g	4 oz
½ cup	*carrot, sliced*	75 g	3 oz
½ cup	*green pepper, seeded, cored and diced*	75 g	3 oz
½ cup	*celery, chopped*	50 g	2 oz
1¾ cups	*cucumber, diced*	250 g	9 oz
1 cup	*low-calorie Italian or French dressing*	225 ml	8 fl oz

Combine the cauliflower, carrot, green pepper, celery and cucumber in a large bowl. Add the dressing and toss to mix well, making sure all the vegetable pieces are well coated. Cover and refrigerate for at least 8 hours, mixing the salad once or twice during that time. One hour before serving, transfer the mixture to a colander placed over a large bowl and drain away the excess dressing. (Pour the excess dressing into a screw-top jar to save for another use.)
* This salad will keep for up to 5 days stored in the refrigerator.

Apple Celery and Raisin Salad

Serves 4

*160 calories
per serving*

2 cups	*apple, cored and diced*	225 g	8 oz
¼ cup	*celery, chopped*	25 g	1 oz
4 tbls	*seedless raisins*	40 g	1½ oz
½ tsp	*ground cinnamon*	½ tsp	½ tsp
2 cups	*plain low-fat yoghurt*	450 g	1 lb

Put the apple, celery and raisins into a bowl. Blend the cinnamon with the yogurt, add to the bowl and toss the ingredients together. Chill well before serving.

Confetti Cottage Cheese

Serves 4

95 calories
per serving

2 cups	low-fat cottage cheese	450 g	1 lb
4 tsp	onion, finely chopped	4 tsp	4 tsp
4 tsp	carrot, finely chopped	4 tsp	4 tsp
4 tsp	green pepper, seeded, cored and finely chopped	4 tsp	4 tsp
¼ tsp	paprika	¼ tsp	4 tsp

Put the cottage cheese into a bowl and add the chopped onion, carrot and green pepper. Mix together well. Divide the mixture between 4 plates and sprinkle each serving with paprika.

* For a more substantial salad, spoon the mixture into the center of 4 small tomatoes which have been cut into 4 sections, nearly to the base. Add 25 calories per serving.

Beet and Onion Salad

Serves 4

25 calories
per serving

1	medium onion, thickly sliced into rings	1	1
2 cups	beets, cooked, peeled and sliced	350 g	12 oz
¼ cup	cider vinegar	60 ml	2 fl oz
	sugar substitute equivalent to 4 tsp sugar		
1 tsp	mixed pickling spices	1 tsp	1 tsp

Put the onion rings and beets into a bowl. Mix the vinegar and sugar substitute, then stir in the vegetables. Tie the pickling spices in a cheesecloth bag and add to the mixture. Cover the bowl and refrigerate for at least 3 hours. Discard the bag of spices before serving.

MEAT

Chili Con Carne

Serves 4

*100 calories
per serving*

6 oz	*lean ground beef*	175 g	6 oz
2 cups	*button mushrooms, sliced*	175 g	6 oz
¼ cup	*onion, chopped*	40 g	1½ oz
¼ cup	*green pepper, cored, seeded, chopped*	40 g	1½ oz
1½ tsp	*chili powder, unsalted*	1½ tsp	1½ tsp
1½ tsp	*dried parsley*	1½ tsp	1½ tsp
½ tsp	*dried oregano*	½ tsp	½ tsp
⅛ tsp	*garlic powder*	⅛ tsp	⅛ tsp
1 pinch	*pepper*	1 pinch	1 pinch
3 cups	*tomato juice, unsalted*	700 ml	1¼ pt

Brown the beef in a large saucepan, using no fat. Drain well in a colander lined with a paper towel to remove as much fat as possible; set aside. Put the mushrooms, onion and green pepper in the pan and cook gently until soft (no need to add liquid). Stir in the beef, seasonings and tomato juice. Simmer for 30 to 40 minutes.

*In place of tomato juice, you can substitute 6 oz/175 g unsalted tomato paste mixed with 2¼ cups/525 ml/18 fl oz water.

Topsy-Turvy Pizza

Serves 4

280 calories
per serving

1 lb	lean ground beef	450 g	1 lb
1/3 cup	cornflakes, crushed	25 g	1 oz
2	egg whites	2	2
1/4 tsp	garlic powder	1/4 tsp	1/4 tsp
1/4 tsp	onion powder	1/4 tsp	1/4 tsp
2 oz	tomato paste, unsalted	50 g	2 oz
1/3 cup	water	75 ml	2½ fl oz
1/8 tsp	dried oregano	1/8 tsp	1/8 tsp
1/8 tsp	black pepper	1/8 tsp	1/8 tsp
2/3 cup	green pepper, seeded, cored, diced	125 g	4 oz
2/3 cup	button mushrooms, sliced	50 g	2 oz
1¾ oz	mozzarella cheese, grated	50 g	1¾ oz
4 tsp	Parmesan cheese, grated	4 tsp	4 tsp

Mix together the beef, cornflakes, egg whites and 1/8 tsp each of the garlic powder and onion powder. Pat the mixture into an 8-in/20-cm pizza pan or similar shallow pan. In a saucepan, blend the tomato paste, water, the remaining garlic powder and onion powder, the oregano and black pepper; simmer for 10 minutes. Meanwhile, sauté the green pepper and mushrooms for 5 minutes in a non-stick pan (or a pan coated with non-stick spray). Spread the sauce over the meat and arrange the cooked vegetables on top. Bake the pizza at 400F/200C/Gas 6 for 20 minutes, then sprinkle with the mozzarella and Parmesan cheeses. Bake for a further 5 minutes to melt the cheese.

* Soy sauce may be added, but only a small amount. Although the calories in 1 tbsp are negligible, the sodium is 1000 mg.
* In place of the vegetables given above, you may substitute similar amounts of any sliced low-calorie vegetables, such as mushrooms, green peppers, broccoli and Chinese pea pods.
* You can vary the basic recipe by substituting 1 lb/450 g/1 lb fresh pork or boned chicken for the beef. Calories per serving change to 215 for the chicken mixture.
* For a change from the traditional rice, serve over a 5-oz/150-g baked potato instead (90 calories).

Gingered Beef with Rice

Serves 4

*420 calories
per serving*

1 lb	*stewing beef*	450 g	1 lb
1 cup	*onions, chopped*	175 g	6 oz
1	*garlic clove, crushed*	1	1
2 tsp	*ground ginger*	2 tsp	2 tsp
1 tsp	*salt*	1 tsp	1 tsp
3 tbls	*vegetable oil*	3 tbls	3 tbls
1 cup	*canned tomatoes, unsalted, chopped*	225 g	8 oz
10 oz	*can of condensed onion soup*	275 g	10 oz
⅔ cup	*rice*	125 g	4½ oz

Remove all visible fat from the beef. Cut the meat into strips and place in a bowl with the onions, garlic, ginger and salt. Mix well and let stand for at least 1 hour. Heat the oil in a large non-stick pan (or one coated with non-stick spray) and sauté this mixture until the meat browns. Add the chopped tomatoes and juice and the condensed onion soup; stir to mix. Bring to the boil, cover and reduce the heat to simmer; cook slowly for 1½ to 2 hours, adding a little water if the mixture seems to be getting too dry. Meanwhile, cook the rice as directed on the packet to be ready at the same time as the beef. Serve the gingered beef over the hot rice.

Enchilada Casserole

315 calories per serving

10 oz	lean ground beef	275 g	10 oz
⅔ cup	onion, chopped	125 g	4 oz
1½ cups	canned tomatoes, unsalted, chopped	275 g	10 oz
2 tsp	chili powder, unsalted	2 tsp	2 tsp
¾ tsp	ground cumin	¾ tsp	¾ tsp
4 oz	Cheddar cheese, grated	125 g	4 oz
4	corn tortillas	4	4

Brown the meat with the onion, using no fat. Drain well in a colander lined with a paper towel to remove as much fat as possible. Return the meat and onion to the pan. Add the tomatoes and juice, chili powder and cumin and mix well. Cut each tortilla into six wedges. Spread the meat mixture into a baking dish or individual-size casseroles sprayed with non-stick spray. Top with the tortilla wedges and sprinkle the cheese over. Bake for 30 minutes at 350F/180C/Gas 4.

*Instead of beef, you can substitute 9 oz/250 g cooked diced chicken. Steam the onions, add to the chicken and proceed as directed.

Stuffed Cabbage Leaves

Serves 4

205 calories
per serving

8	large cabbage leaves	8	8
1 lb	lean ground beef	450 g	1 lb
¼ cup	onion, chopped	40 g	1½ oz
½ cup	cooked rice	100 g	3½ oz
⅓ cup	green peppers, seeded, cored, chopped	50 g	2 oz
½ cup	button mushrooms, sliced	40 g	1½ oz
1 tbls	fresh parsley, chopped	1 tbls	1 tbls
1 tsp	garlic powder	1 tsp	1 tsp
1 tbls	Worcestershire sauce	1 tbls	1 tbls
1 cup	Basic Tomato Sauce (see page 154)	225 ml	8 fl oz

Parboil the cabbage leaves in unsalted water until they are just limp; drain and set aside. Brown the meat with the onion, using no fat. Drain well in a colander lined with paper towel to remove as much fat as possible. Return the meat and onion to the pan. Add the cooked rice, green pepper, mushrooms, fresh parsley and garlic powder and mix well. Mix in the Worcestershire sauce. Divide the mixture into 8 portions. Roll up each portion inside a cabbage leaf, folding over both ends to enclose the filling. Place the cabbage rolls side by side in a non-stick baking pan or shallow casserole and pour the tomato sauce over them. Cover with foil and bake for 30 to 40 minutes at 350F/180C/Gas 4.

Chinese Beef and Vegetables

Serves 4 *265 calories*
per serving
(plus 100 calories for ½ cup/100 g/3½ oz cooked rice)

2 tbls	reduced-calorie Italian dressing	2 tbls	2 tbls
1 tbls	lemon juice	1 tbls	1 tbls
1 tbls	vinegar	1 tbls	1 tbls
4 tsp	cornstarch	4 tsp	4 tsp
1 cup	unsalted stock	225 ml	8 fl oz
4 tsp	vegetable oil	4 tsp	4 tsp
¼ tsp	ground ginger	¼ tsp	¼ tsp
¼ tsp	garlic powder	¼ tsp	¼ tsp
1 lb	lean beef, cut into thin strips	450 g	1 lb
2 cups	mixed Chinese vegetables	375 g	13 oz
2 cups	green beans cut into 1-in/2.5-cm pieces	275 g	10 oz

* If you use canned beans, drain and rinse them.

Twelve to 24 hours before cooking, marinate the meat in a mixture of the reduced-calorie dressing, lemon juice and vinegar; cover and refrigerate until needed.

Dissolve the cornstarch in the stock. Heat the oil in a large frying pan or wok. Add the vegetables and stir-fry for 3 minutes. Stir the cornstarch mixture and pour it into the pan. Continue cooking, stirring until all the ingredients are well mixed and the liquid has thickened, about 3 minutes more. Serve with rice.

Dinner in a Tater

Serves 4

360 calories per serving

4 (5 oz each)	potatoes	4 (150 g each)	4 (5 oz each)
1 lb	lean ground beef	450 g	1 lb
1 cup	carrots, thinly sliced	150 g	5 oz
1 cup	green beans, trimmed and sliced	175 g	6 oz
1 cup	zucchini, thinly sliced	150 g	5 oz
3 tbls	onion, chopped	3 tbls	3 tbls
1/8 tsp	salt	1/8 tsp	1/8 tsp
to taste	black pepper	to taste	to taste
1 cup	plain low-fat yoghurt	225 ml	8 fl oz
4	lemon or lime wedges	4	4

Scrub the potatoes and bake them at 400F/200C/Gas 6 until soft. Meanwhile, brown the meat in a non-stick pan, using no fat. Drain well in a colander lined with a paper towel to remove as much fat as possible. Set aside. In the same pan, lightly sauté the carrots, beans, zucchini and onions until tender but still crisp. Mix them into the meat and season with the salt and pepper. Keep the mixture warm until the potatoes are done. Cut a large cross in the top of each potato. Press the sides firmly to open them. Spoon a quarter of the warm meat and vegetable mixture over each potato and top with a quarter of the yoghurt. Garnish with the lemon or lime wedges on the side.

Quick Beef Stroganoff

Serves 4

290 calories
per serving
(plus 100 calories for ½ cup/100 g/3½ oz cooked rice or noodles)

1¼ lb	*beef fillet*	575 g	1¼ lb
1 tbls	*margarine*	15 g	½ oz
¼ cup	*onions, chopped*	40 g	1½ oz
1 cup	*button mushrooms, sliced*	75 g	3 oz
1 cup	*beef consommé*	225 ml	8 fl oz
½ cup	*plain low-fat yoghurt*	125 ml	4 fl oz

Remove all visible fat from the beef. Pound the meat with a mallet or rolling pin until about ¼ in/5 mm thick, then cut it into strips. Melt the margarine in a large frying pan and sauté the onions and mushrooms. Add the beef strips and brown them quickly. Remove the beef mixture and keep it warm. Add the consommé to the pan and simmer for 10 minutes to reduce the volume slightly. Return the beef mixture to the pan and add the yoghurt. Heat through, stirring, but do not let the sauce boil or it will curdle. Serve immediately over rice or noodles.

Notes

Marinated Flank Steak

Serves 4

180 calories
per serving

½ cup	reduced-calorie Italian dressing	125 ml	4 fl oz
2 tbls	lemon juice	2 tbls	2 tbls
2 tbls	vinegar	2 tbls	2 tbls
¼ tsp	garlic powder	¼ tsp	¼ tsp
4 (4 oz)	lean steaks	4 (125 g)	4 (4 oz)

Mix the Italian dressing, lemon juice, vinegar and garlic powder in a shallow dish. Place the meat in the marinade, turn once, cover and refrigerate for 24 to 48 hours. Turn occasionally during this time. Broil or grill on a high heat until the steaks are cooked the way you like them, 3 to 5 minutes per side. Slice thinly across the grain of the meat.

* Marinated chicken breasts are just as tasty. Use 4 breast pieces weighing 4 oz/125 g each, for 150 calories per serving.

Beef Loaf

Serves 4

220 calories
per serving

1 lb	lean ground beef	450 g	1 lb
¼ cup	oatmeal	25 g	1 oz
2	egg whites	2	2
½ cup	canned tomatoes, unsalted, chopped	125 g	4 oz
¼ cup	onion, chopped	40 g	1½ oz
¼ cup	green pepper, seeded, cored, chopped	40 g	1½ oz
¼ cup	carrot, chopped	40 g	1½ oz
¼ tsp	garlic powder	¼ tsp	¼ tsp
¼ tsp	dried basil	¼ tsp	¼ tsp

Mix all the ingredients together thoroughly and divide into 4 individual-size loaf pans or casseroles. Bake for 1 hour at 350F/180C/Gas 4. There's no need to drain the loaves before serving if lean meat has been used (the juices are low in fat and will add moisture and flavor).

*To ensure leanness, buy the beef as whole steaks, trim off all visible fat and grind it yourself.

Swedish Meatballs Stroganoff

Serves 4

310 calories
per serving

(plus 100 calories for ½ cup/100 g/3½ oz cooked rice or noodles)

¼ cup	skim milk	4 tbls	4 tbls
1	egg	1	1
2 tbls	onion, finely chopped	2 tbls	2 tbls
1½	bread slices, finely crumbled	1½	1½
12 oz	lean ground beef	350 g	12 oz

Sauce

1 tbls	margarine	15 g	½ oz
½ cup	onion, chopped	75 g	3 oz
2 tbls	flour	2 tbls	2 tbls
2 cups	unsalted stock	475 ml	16 fl oz
2 tbls	low-calorie catsup	2 tbls	2 tbls
¼ cup	plain low-fat yoghurt	4 tbls	4 tbls

In a large bowl, beat together the milk and egg; add the onion and crumbled bread and let the mixture stand for 5 minutes. Add the ground beef and mix thoroughly. Divide the mixture into 24 equal pieces and shape them into small balls. Place them slightly apart in a non-stick pan and bake for 20 to 30 minutes at 375F/190C/Gas 5. Meanwhile, make the sauce. Melt the margarine in a large frying pan. Add the onion and cook until transparent. Sprinkle the flour over and cook for 2 minutes, stirring. Add the stock and catsup and simmer over low heat, stirring constantly, until the mixture starts simmering. Add the cooked meatballs and heat them through, then add the yoghurt and heat for another 1 or 2 minutes until the sauce returns to simmering. (Do not let it boil or the sauce will curdle.) Serve over rice or noodles.

Fajitas

Serves 4

400 calories
per serving

1 lb	Marinated Steak, sliced (see page 112)	450 g	1 lb
8	corn tortillas	8	8
2 cups	Barbecue Sauce (see page 155)	475 ml	16 fl oz

Make the marinated flank steak, as in the recipe on page 000; slice the meat and keep it warm. Heat the tortillas in a 300F/150C/Gas 2 oven until warm, about 10 to 15 minutes. Put equal amounts of sliced meat on each tortilla and pour the barbecue sauce over the meat. Fold the tortillas around the steak and serve warm, two to each person.

*This Mexican dish (pronounced far-hee-tahs) is a favorite in Texas.

Spaghetti Casserole

Serves 4

380 calories
per serving

½ lb	spaghetti	225 g	8 oz
10 oz	lean ground beef	275 g	10 oz
6 cups	Basic Tomato Sauce (see page 154)	1.4 L	2⅓ pt
2 tbls	Parmesan cheese, grated	2 tbls	2 tbls

Cook the spaghetti in boiling unsalted water for about 10 minutes, or until it is 'al dente'. Rinse it under cold running water to remove some of the starch, then rinse again under hot water, drain and set aside. Brown the beef in a large frying pan, using no fat. Drain well in a colander lined with a paper towel to remove as much fat as possible. Return the meat to the pan, add the tomato sauce and mix well. Coat a medium-size casserole with non-stick spray. Put the spaghetti in the bottom and stir in the meat sauce and 1 tbls of the Parmesan cheese. Sprinkle the remaining 1 tbls Parmesan on top. Cover and bake for 30 minutes at 350F/180C/Gas 4.

Spaghetti with Meat Sauce

Serves 4

335 calories per serving

18 oz	*lean ground beef*	525 g	18 oz
⅓ cup	*onion, chopped*	50g	2 oz
⅓ cup	*green pepper, seeded, cored, chopped*	50 g	2 oz
8 oz	*tomato paste, unsalted*	225 g	8 oz
1 cup	*water*	225 ml	8 fl oz
2 tsp	*dried parsley*	2 tsp	2 tsp
½ tsp	*dried oregano*	½ tsp	½ tsp
¼ tsp	*dried thyme*	¼ tsp	¼ tsp
¼ tsp	*rosemary, crumbled*	¼ tsp	¼ tsp
¼ tsp	*dried basil*	¼ tsp	¼ tsp
¼ tsp	*garlic powder*	¼ tsp	¼ tsp
1 pinch	*pepper*	1 pinch	1 pinch
1	*bay leaf*	1	1
¼ lb	*spaghetti*	125 g	4 oz

Brown the meat with the onion and green pepper, using no fat. Drain well in a colander lined with a paper towel to remove as much fat as possible. Return the meat mixture to the pan. Add the tomato paste, water, seasonings and bay leaf. Mix well, cover and simmer for 30 minutes. (If the sauce gets too thick during this time, add a little more water.) Meanwhile, cook the pasta in unsalted boiling water until it is just 'al dente'; drain well.

Stuffed Peppers

Serves 4

300 calories
per serving

1 lb	lean ground beef	450 g	1 lb
½ cup	onion, chopped	75 g	3 oz
2 cups	cooked rice	200 g	14 oz
½ cup	Basic Tomato Sauce (see page 154)	125 ml	4 fl oz
4	small green peppers, seeded, cored, blanched	4	4

Brown the meat with the onion, using no fat. Drain well in a colander lined with a paper towel to remove as much fat as possible. Combine with the cooked rice and the tomato sauce. Put one-quarter of the mixture into each green pepper. Place in a baking dish and bake uncovered for 25 minutes at 350F/180C/Gas 4. Add a little extra tomato sauce, if desired.
*If using already cooked beef, reduce the amount to 12 oz/350 g.
*Alternatively, leave out the beef and use 12 oz/350 g tuna or cooked chicken or turkey.

Stir-Fry Vegetables and Beef

Serves 4

195 calories
per serving
(plus 100 calories for ½ cup/100 g/3½ oz cooked rice)

1 tbls	vegetable oil	1 tbls	1 tbls
½ lb	steak cut into thin strips	225 g	8 oz
2 cups	button mushrooms, sliced	175 g	6 oz
4	medium broccoli stalks, chopped	4	4
1 cup	green pepper, seeded, cored, chopped	175 g	6 oz
1 cup	Chinese pea pods	150 g	5 oz
4	green onions, chopped	4	4

Heat the oil in a large frying pan or wok. Add the beef and stir-fry over a medium-high heat for about 10 minutes. Add the remaining ingredients and stir-fry for about 15 minutes, or until the vegetables are tender but still crisp. Serve alone or over rice.

Beef Stroganoff

Serves 4

*380 calories
per serving*
(plus 100 calories per ½ cup/100 g/3½ oz cooked rice or noodles)

2 lb	*round or flank steak*	900 g	2 lb
2 tbls	*margarine*	25 g	1 oz
½ cup	*onions, chopped*	75 g	3 oz
½ cup	*small button mushrooms*	40 g	1½ oz
2 tbls	*tomato paste, unsalted*	2 tbls	2 tbls
1 cup	*unsalted stock*	225 ml	8 fl oz
1 tsp	*mustard powder*	1 tsp	1 tsp
2 tbls	*Worcestershire sauce*	2 tbls	2 tbls
1 tsp	*black pepper*	1 tsp	1 tsp
1	*bay leaf*	1	1
1 tbls	*flour*	1 tbls	1 tbls
2 tbls	*water*	2 tbls	2 tbls
¾ cup	*plain low-fat yoghurt*	175 ml	6 fl oz

Remove all visible fat from the steak. Cut the meat into finger-size strips. Melt half the margarine in a non-stick frying pan. Add the meat and fry, stirring, until the pieces are brown on all sides. Remove the meat from the pan and set aside. Sauté the onions in the remaining pan juices until golden. Remove the onions and put them with the meat. Add the remaining margarine to the pan and sauté the mushrooms until almost tender. Return the meat and onions to the pan. In a bowl, combine the tomato paste, stock, mustard, Worcestershire sauce and black pepper. Stir this into the meat mixture and add the bay leaf. Heat the mixture to simmering, cover and cook gently for 30 minutes or longer, until the meat is tender. Remove the bay leaf. Make a smooth paste of the flour and water and stir it into the meat mixture. Cook over low heat, stirring, until the mixture thickens. Add the yoghurt and heat through. (Do not let it boil or the sauce will curdle.) Serve alone or with rice or noodles.

POULTRY

Sautéed Chicken Breasts

Serves 4

275 calories
per serving

1½ lb	boneless chicken breasts, skinned	675 g	1½ lb
1½ tbls	margarine	1½ tbls	1½ tbls
⅜ cup	dry sherry or white wine	6 tbls	6 tbls
¾-½ tsp	dried basil or tarragon	¾-½ tsp	¾-½ tsp
¼ tsp	white pepper	¼ tsp	¼ tsp
¼ tsp	paprika	¼ tsp	¼ tsp
	fresh parsley, finely chopped, to taste		

Place each chicken breast between 2 pieces of wax paper. Pound with a wooden mallet, rolling pin or other suitable utensil to a thickness of ½ in (15 mm). Melt the margarine in a non-stick pan over medium to medium-high heat. Add the pounded chicken pieces. Sauté on one side until brown, about 4 to 5 minutes. Turn the chicken over. Add the sherry and let it come to the boil so the alcohol evaporates (eliminating most of the sherry's calories but leaving the flavor). Sprinkle the spices over the chicken pieces. Cook another 4 to 5 minutes. Do not overcook or the tender texture and flavor of the meat may be affected. Sprinkle with the fresh parsley and serve.

* This is an elegant, easy, quick and protein-rich recipe. In addition, the margarine provides some polyunsaturated fat.

Chicken Curry Casserole

Serves 4

*350 calories
per serving*

2 cups	boneless cooked chicken, diced	350 g	12 oz
2 cups	cooked rice	400 g	14 oz
1⅓ cups	green pepper, seeded, cored, chopped	225 g	8 oz
6	green onions, chopped (including tops)	6	6
12	large mushrooms, sliced	12	12
1½ cups	unsalted chicken stock	350 ml	12 fl oz
1 tbls	curry powder	1 tbls	1 tbls
1 tsp	cornstarch	1 tsp	1 tsp

Coat the casserole dish with non-stick spray. In a large bowl, mix together the chicken pieces, cooked rice, green peppers, onions and mushrooms. Blend together the stock, curry powder and cornstarch, pour this over the chicken mixture and stir to mix thoroughly. Transfer the mixture to the casserole. Bake for 45 minutes at 350F/180C/Gas 4.

* When cooked chicken is called for in a recipe, bake it in the oven at 350F/180C/Gas 4 until it is cooked. Chicken that is oven-baked can be reheated without getting tough.

* This recipe can be prepared up to 2 days in advance. When all the ingredients have been mixed and transferred to the casserole, cover the dish with plastic wrap and refrigerate until needed. Bake as directed.

Broccoli Rice with Chicken Liver

Serves 4

360 calories per serving

3 tbls	*margarine*	40 g	1½ oz
1 lb	*chicken livers*	450 g	1 lb
¼ cup	*onion, chopped*	40 g	1½ oz
2 cups	*broccoli, chopped*	200 g	7 oz
1 tsp	*dried parsley*	1 tsp	1 tsp
2 cups	*cooked rice*	400 g	14 oz
¾ cup	*unsalted chicken stock*	175 ml	6 fl oz

Melt the margarine in a non-stick pan and cook the chicken livers thoroughly. Add the onion, broccoli and parsley and cook over a medium heat for 5 minutes, stirring occasionally. Coat a casserole with non-stick spray. Spread the cooked rice and add the liver mixture. Pour the chicken stock over and bake, uncovered, for 30 minutes at 350F/180C/Gas 4.

* This dish can be prepared a day ahead. After adding the stock, cover the casserole and refrigerate until needed. Bake covered, for 20 minutes, then a further 20 minutes uncovered.

Spanish Chicken

Serves 4

325 calories
per serving

4	chicken breasts	4	4
1 tsp	paprika	1 tsp	1 tsp
2 tbls	butter or margarine	25 g	1 oz
¼ cup	onion, chopped	40 g	1½ oz
½ cup	green pepper, seeded, cored, chopped	75 g	3 oz
½ cup	carrots, chopped	50 g	2 oz
½ cup	celery, chopped	65 g	2½ oz
1	garlic clove, minced	1	1
1½ cups	tomato juice, unsalted	350 ml	12 fl oz
¾ cup	button mushrooms, sliced	75 g	2½ oz
1-2 tbls	flour	1-2 tbls	1-2 tbls

Rinse and dry the chicken breasts and sprinkle the paprika over them. Place them in a non-stick casserole dish or one that has been coated with non-stick spray. Melt the butter or margarine in a saucepan and sauté the onion, green pepper, carrots, celery and garlic for 15 minutes. Add the tomato juice then pour the mixture over the chicken breasts. Bake uncovered at 350F/ 180C/Gas 4 for 50 minutes. Remove from the oven, stir in the sliced mushrooms and continue baking for another 10 minutes. To thicken the sauce before serving, blend the flour with a little water until smooth and pour this into the sauce, stirring well. Simmer for 3 minutes, stirring frequently.

Curried Chicken and Rice

Serves 4

300 calories per serving

¼ cup	*raw bran*	4 tbls	4 tbls
1 tsp	*paprika*	1 tsp	1 tsp
1 tsp	*curry powder*	1 tsp	1 tsp
¼ tsp	*dried thyme*	¼ tsp	¼ tsp
⅛ tsp	*pepper*	⅛ tsp	⅛ tsp
4 (4 oz)	*boneless chicken pieces, skinned*	4 (125 g)	4 (4 oz)
½ cup	*onions, chopped*	75 g	3 oz
⅛ tsp	*garlic powder*	⅛ tsp	⅛ tsp
⅛ tsp	*ground ginger*	⅛ tsp	⅛ tsp
1⅓ cups	*water*	315 ml	11 fl oz
⅔ cup	*brown rice*	125 g	4½ oz
⅛ tsp	*ground turmeric*	⅛ tsp	⅛ tsp

Combine the bran, paprika, curry powder, thyme and pepper in a paper or plastic bag. Place the chicken pieces in a bag, one at a time, and shake well to coat; shake off excess bran mixture while removing the meat from the bag. Heat 2 to 4 tbls water in a large frying pan until boiling. Add the chicken, cover and steam for 10 minutes on each side. (Add more water during steaming if necessary.) Remove the chicken pieces from the pan. Add the onions, garlic powder and ginger to the leftover juices; cover and steam until the onions are soft. Add the measured water and heat to boiling. Meanwhile, put the rice and turmeric into a casserole. Pour the boiling mixture over, mix thoroughly and arrange the chicken pieces on top. Cover with a lid or foil and bake for 1 hour at 350F/180C/Gas 4.

Baked Chicken Parmesan

Serves 4

*230 calories
per serving*

2½ tbls	*cornflakes, crushed*	2½ tbls	2½ tbls
2½ tbls	*Parmesan cheese, grated*	2½ tbls	2½ tbls
1½ tbls	*dried parsley*	1½ tbls	1½ tbls
¼ tsp	*poultry seasoning*	¼ tsp	¼ tsp
⅛ tsp	*onion powder*	⅛ tsp	⅛ tsp
1 pinch	*garlic powder*	1 pinch	1 pinch
4 (4 oz)	*boneless chicken pieces, skinned*	4 (125 g)	4 (4 oz)

In a small bowl, mix together all the ingredients except the chicken. Place the chicken in a baking pan. Sprinkle about 1 tbls of cornflake mixture over each serving of chicken. Turn the meat over and repeat. Dust with paprika for extra color. Bake for 45 to 60 minutes at 375F/190C/Gas 5.

Lemon Chicken

Serves 4

*150 calories
per serving*

½ cup	*lemon juice*	125 ml	4 fl oz
½ tsp	*pepper*	½ tsp	½ tsp
¼ tsp	*mustard powder*	¼ tsp	¼ tsp
¼ tsp	*paprika*	¼ tsp	¼ tsp
¼ tsp	*dried thyme*	¼ tsp	¼ tsp
¼ tsp	*curry powder*	¼ tsp	4 tsp
4 (4 oz)	*boneless chicken pieces, skinned*	4 (125 g)	4 (4 oz)

Place the lemon juice and seasonings in a baking dish and beat with a fork. Add the chicken, cover and refrigerate for 8 to 12 hours. Turn the meat at least once while it marinates. Bake uncovered until tender, about 1 hour, at 350F/180C/Gas 4, basting with the pan juices. (The chicken will brown only slightly.)

Chicken Oriental

Serves 4
270 calories
per serving
(plus 100 calories for ½ cup/100 g/3½ oz cooked rice)

4 tsp	cornstarch	4 tsp	4 tsp
1 cup	pineapple juice	225 ml	8 fl oz
4 tsp	vegetable oil	4 tsp	4 tsp
1 lb	boneless chicken, skinned and diced	450 g	1 lb
½ cup	pineapple chunks, canned in juice	75 g	3 oz
1 cup	bean sprouts	65 g	2½ oz
1 cup	celery, diagonally sliced	125 g	4 oz
1 cup	green pepper, seeded, cored, sliced	125 g	4 oz
1 cup	onion, diced	175 g	6 oz

Dissolve the cornstarch in the pineapple juice; set aside. Heat the oil in a large frying pan or wok. Add the chicken and stir-fry over a medium-high heat until cooked through. Remove the meat and keep warm. Add the pineapple chunks and vegetables to the oil and meat juices remaining in the pan and stir-fry for 3 to 4 minutes. Return the chicken to the pan, stir in the cornstarch mixture and pour it into the pan. Bring to the boil stirring quickly to coat the chicken and vegetables while the mixture thickens. Serve at once over rice.

* Soy sauce may be added, but only a small amount. Although the calories in 1 tbls are negligible, the sodium is 1000 mg.

* In place of those given above, you may substitute a similar amount of any sliced low-calorie vegetables.

* You can vary the basic recipe by substituting 1 lb/450 g lean beef or pork or raw, peeled deveined shrimp for the chicken. Calories per serving change to 300 for the beef or pork mixture, 225 for the shrimp mixture.

Turkey or Chicken Stuffing

Serves 4

65 calories
per serving

½ cup	carrots, chopped	75 g	3 oz
½ cup	celery, chopped	65 g	2½ oz
½ cup	mushrooms, chopped	25 g	1 oz
½ cup	onion, chopped	75 g	3 oz
2 cups	unsalted stock	475 ml	16 fl oz
1 tsp	dried parsley	1 tsp	1 tsp
½ tsp	poultry seasoning	½ tsp	½ tsp
¼ tsp	garlic powder	¼ tsp	¼ tsp
¼ tsp	paprika	¼ tsp	¼ tsp
1 cup	bean sprouts	65 g	2½ oz
2	bread slices, cubed	2	2

Put the carrots, celery, mushrooms, onion and stock into a saucepan, add the parsley, poultry seasoning, garlic powder and paprika. Cook for about 15 minutes or until the vegetables are tender and the stock has reduced. Add the bean sprouts and bread cubes. Toss to mix well. Coat a casserole dish with non-stick spray, spoon in the vegetable mixture and press down firmly. Bake for 30 minutes at 350F/180C/Gas 4 until light brown. Serve with sliced turkey, as a substitute for the traditional turkey stuffing.

Chicken of Five Seasonings

Serves 4

*300 calories
per serving*

2 tbls	*flour*	2 tbls	2 tbls
½ tsp	*dried parsley*	½ tsp	½ tsp
¼ tsp	*dried thyme*	¼ tsp	¼ tsp
¼ tsp	*dried oregano*	¼ tsp	¼ tsp
¼ tsp	*rosemary, crumbled*	¼ tsp	¼ tsp
¼ tsp	*pepper*	¼ tsp	¼ tsp
4 (4 oz)	*boneless chicken pieces, skinned*	4 (125 g)	4 (4 oz)
½ cup	*onion, chopped*	75 g	3 oz
½ cup	*button mushrooms, sliced*	40 g	1½ oz
4	*tomatoes, chopped*	4	4
1 tbls	*lemon juice*	1 tbls	1 tbls
⅔ cup	*brown rice*	125 g	4½ oz

Combine the flour, herbs and pepper in a paper or plastic bag. Place the chicken pieces in the bag, one at a time, and shake well to coat. Remove the chicken, reserving the seasoned flour. Heat 2 to 4 tbls water in a large frying pan until boiling. Add the chicken, cover and steam for 10 minutes on each side. (Add more water during steaming if necessary.) Remove the chicken pieces from the pan and add the onions, mushrooms, tomatoes, lemon juice and leftover seasoned flour. Cover and steam until the vegetables are just tender. Transfer the vegetables to a large measuring cup. Add water up to 1⅔ cup/400 ml/14 fl oz mark and put this mixture on to boil. Meanwhile, put the uncooked rice in a casserole. Pour the boiling mixture over, mix thoroughly and arrange the chicken pieces on top. Cover with a lid or foil and bake for 1 hour at 350F/180C/Gas 4.

Chicken Tetrazzini

Serves 4

*380 calories
per serving*

¼ lb	noodles	25 g	4 oz
1 lb	boneless cooked chicken, diced	450 g	1 lb
10 fl oz	can of condensed mushroom soup	300 ml	10 fl oz
¾ cup	green pepper, seeded, cored, sliced	125 g	4½ oz
2 tsp	dried parsley	2 tsp	2 tsp
2 tsp	paprika	2 tsp	2 tsp
	black pepper, to taste		

Cook the noodles for 10 minutes in unsalted water, or until they are 'al dente'; drain, rinse and drain again well. Coat a casserole with non-stick spray. In a large bowl, combine the noodles, diced chicken, condensed soup, green pepper, parsley, paprika and black pepper; mix well and pour into the casserole. Sprinkle the top with extra paprika for color. Bake, covered, for 45 minutes at 350F/180C/Gas 4.

Stuffed Chicken Breasts

Serves 4

*300 calories
per serving*

4 (4oz)	boneless chicken breast pieces, skinned	4 (125 g)	4 (4 oz)
8 slices	reduced-calorie cheese	8 slices	8 slices
9 oz	green beans	9 oz	9 oz
2 tbls	pimento, seeded, cored, chopped	2 tbls	2 tbls
1 cup	Tomato Sauce (see page 154)	225 ml	8 fl oz

Pound the chicken pieces between sheets of wax paper until about ½ in/15 mm thick. Top each piece with two slices of cheese and one quarter of the mixed green beans and pimento. Bring the ends of each chicken piece together and secure with a wooden cocktail stick. Place in a baking dish, smooth side up, and pour the tomato sauce over. Cover and bake for 20 minutes at 350F/180C/Gas 4. Uncover and continue baking for another 20 minutes.

Barbeque Chicken

Serves 4

*340 calories
per serving*

2 (1½ lb)	small chickens	2 (275 g)	2 (1½ lb)
3 tbls	paprika	3 tbls	3 tbls
2 cups	Barbecue Sauce (see page 155)	475 ml	16 fl oz

Halve the chickens and remove the skin. Sprinkle them with the paprika and place them in a baking pan coated with non-stick spray. Cover the pan with foil and bake for 45 minutes at 350F/ 180C/Gas 4. Remove the foil cover and spread the barbecue sauce over the chicken halves. Return them to the oven and continue baking, uncovered, for 15 minutes more.

FISH

Foil-Baked Fish

Serves 4

*235 calories
per serving*

2 lb	*lean fish, cleaned and washed*	900 g	2 lb
	skim milk, to soak		
1 cup	*button mushrooms, sliced*	75 g	3 oz
½ cup	*carrots, sliced*	65 g	2½ oz
½ cup	*green pepper, seeded, cored, sliced*	50 g	2 oz
½ cup	*onion, diced*	75 g	3 oz
½ cup	*celery with leaves, chopped*	65 g	2½ oz
	lemon juice, herbs, paprika, to taste		

Use lean fish, such as haddock, flounder or perch, about 35 cal/1 oz (30 cal/25 g). Soak the fish in skim milk for at least 30 minutes; drain. Divide the fish into four 8-oz/225-g portions. Place each portion on a generous piece of heavy-duty foil and add one-quarter of the vegetables on top. Sprinkle on lemon juice, dried herbs such as parsley and oregano, and paprika to taste. Seal tightly, rolling the foil from the top and sides. Bake for 25 minutes at 450F/230C/Gas 8.

*If you don't have heavy-duty foil, use a double thickness of the ordinary kind.

*This recipe can also be cooked on an outdoor barbecue grill.

Italian Sauced Fish

Serves 4

*255 calories
per serving*

2 lb	lean fish, cleaned and washed	900 g	2 lb
6 oz	tomato paste, unsalted	175 g	6 oz
1 cup	water	225 g	8 fl oz
½ cup	button mushrooms, sliced	40 g	1½ oz
¼ cup	green pepper, seeded, cored, chopped	40 g	1½ oz
¼ cup	onion, chopped	40 g	1½ oz
½ tsp	dried basil	½ tsp	½ tsp
½ tsp	dried oregano	½ tsp	½ tsp
¼ tsp	pepper	¼ tsp	¼ tsp
¼ tsp	garlic powder	¼ tsp	¼ tsp

Use lean fish such as haddock, flounder or perch, about 35 cal/1 oz (30 cal/25 g). Divide the fish into four 8-oz/225-g portions and arrange in a baking dish. Mix the tomato paste and the water in a bowl until smooth; add the vegetables and seasonings. Pour the sauce over the fish. Bake uncovered until the fish flakes easily with a fork, 20-25 minutes, at 350F/180C/Gas 4.

*A little cheese brings an authentic touch to this dish. Before baking, sprinkle the fish pieces with 2 oz/50 g grated mozzarella cheese (adds 40 calories per serving) or stir 4 tbls Parmesan cheese into the sauce (an extra 30 calories per serving).

Shrimp Louisianne

3 tbls	*margarine*	40 g	3 tbls
½ medium	*onion, chopped*	½ medium	½ medium
2 stalks	*celery, chopped*	2 stalks	2 stalks
½ medium	*green pepper, chopped*	½ medium	½ medium
¼ cup	*flour*	75 g	3 tbls
2½ cups	*canned tomatoes, chopped*	575 ml	20 fl oz
1	*bay leaf*	1	1
1 tsp	*parsley, chopped*	1 tsp	1 tsp
1 tsp	*Worcestershire sauce*	1 tsp	1 tsp
2 drops	*Tabasco sauce*	2 drops	2 drops
1 lb	*fresh or canned shrimp*	450 g	16 oz
½ cup	*rice (uncooked)*	125 g	4 oz

Melt the margarine in a large pan. Add the onion, celery and pepper and cook for about 20 minutes over low heat until vegetables are limp, and tender. Stir in the flour. Heat until mixture starts to bubble. Add the tomatoes, herbs and sauces. Cover the pan and simmer for about 30 minutes. Add the shrimp and heat thoroughly, about 10 minutes, over low heat, stirring occasionally. Serve over rice.

Bebe's Shrimp with Peppers

Serves 4

162 calories
per serving

(plus 100 calories for ½ cup/100 g/3½ oz cooked rice)

2 tsp	cornstarch	2 tsp	2 tsp
1 tsp	dry sherry	1 tsp	1 tsp
1 tsp	Tabasco pepper sauce	1 tsp	1 tsp
1 lb	peeled shrimp (fresh or thawed)	450 g	1 lb
4 tsp	sesame oil	4 tsp	4 tsp
1	green pepper, cored, seeded, chopped	1	1
1	red pepper, cored, seeded, chopped	1	1
1	garlic clove, crushed	1	1
1 slice	fresh ginger	1 slice	1 slice
2 tbls	water	2 tbls	2 tbls
2	green onions, chopped	2	2

Dissolve 1 tsp of the cornstarch in the sherry and Tabasco; mix into the shrimp and set aside. Heat the oil in a large non-stick frying pan or wok. Add the green and red peppers and stir-fry over a medium heat for about 2 minutes. Remove the peppers and keep warm. Add the ginger slice and garlic clove, fry them for 30 seconds to flavor the oil then discard. Add the shrimp and stir-fry until they are cooked through, about 4 minutes. Return the peppers to the pan. Dissolve the remaining 1 tsp cornstarch in the water and add it to the pan. Bring to the boil, stirring quickly to coat the shrimp and peppers while the liquid thickens. Serve at once over rice, garnished with chopped green onions.

*Rinsed and drained canned shrimp can be used in place of fresh or frozen. Instead of stir-frying them for 5 minutes, you need only to heat them through before adding the cooked peppers.

Tuna Casserole

¼ cup	onion, chopped	40 g	1½ oz
¼ cup	green pepper, seeded, cored, chopped	40 g	1½ oz
¼ cup	pimento, drained and chopped	4 tbls	4 tbls
2 cups	low-fat cottage cheese	450 g	1 lb
8 oz	canned tuna in brine, drained	225 g	8 oz
1 tsp	mixed dried herbs	1 tsp	1 tsp
4	egg whites	4	4

Cook the onion and green pepper until tender but still crisp (steam, or dry-fry without fat in a non-stick pan). Drain well. Thoroughly mix the onion, green pepper, pimento, cottage cheese, tuna and herbs. Beat the egg whites until stiff, then fold them into the mixture. Divide between four individual-size loaf pans or casseroles. Bake uncovered for 30 minutes at 350F/ 180C/Gas 4. Drain off any excess liquid and top each serving with 4 tbls Mushroom Sauce (see page 158).

Broiled Shrimp Paprika

20 large	shrimp or prawns	20 large	20 large
2 tbls	paprika	2 tbls	2 tbls
4 tbls	margarine	4 tbls	4 tbls

Peel shrimp or prawns, leaving the tail on. Split down center, open them out and sprinkle paprika on them. Place on non-stick broiler pan. Melt 2 tbls of margarine and spoon over the shrimps. Broil under medium heat for about 15 minutes. Serve with the rest of the melted margarine.

Scallops Hawaiian

Serves 4

200 calories
per serving

(plus 100 calories for ½ cup/100 g/3½ oz cooked rice)

4 tsp	cornstarch	4 tsp	4 tsp
	brown sugar substitute equivalent to ½ tsp brown sugar		
½ tsp	ground ginger	½ tsp	½ tsp
⅓ cup	canned pineapple juice	75 ml	3 fl oz
1 tsp	vinegar	1 tsp	1 tsp
4 tsp	vegetable oil	4 tsp	4 tsp
1 cup	green pepper, seeded, cored sliced	125 g	4 oz
1 lb	scallops, raw	450 g	1 lb
2 cups	pineapple chunks in own juice	350 g	12 oz

In a small bowl, combine the cornstarch, brown sugar substitute and ginger. Blend the pineapple juice and vinegar. Set aside. Heat the oil in a large pan or wok. Add the green pepper and stir-fry over a medium heat for 2 minutes; remove. Stir-fry the scallops for 2 minutes; remove. Stir the pineapple juice (the cornstarch will have settled) and pour it into the frying pan. When the mixture begins to bubble, stir until it thickens. Add the green pepper, mushrooms and pineapple chunks. Simmer for 2 minutes, mixing to coat in the sauce. Add the scallops and continue simmering for 1 minute. Serve with rice.

*You can used cooked scallops instead of raw, but reduce the amount to 12 oz/350 g; there is no need to stir-fry them.

*Soy sauce may be added, but only a small amount. Although the calories in 1 tbls are negligible, the sodium is 1000 mg.

Company Tuna Casserole

Serves 4

*230 calories
per serving*

2 tbls	*butter or margarine*	25 g	1 oz
2 tbls	*flour*	25 g	1 oz
2 cups	*skim milk*	475 ml	16 fl oz
13 oz	*canned tuna in brine, drained*	375 g	13 oz
¼ cup	*onion, grated*	40 g	1½ oz
2 tbls	*pimento, chopped*	2 tbls	2 tbls
1 tsp	*Worcestershire sauce*	1 tsp	1 tsp
1 pinch	*salt*	1 pinch	1 pinch
3 tbls	*breadcrumbs*	3 tbls	3 tbls
1 tbls	*Parmesan cheese, grated*	1 tbls	1 tbls

Melt the butter or margarine in a saucepan. Add the flour, mix well, and allow to foam for 2 minutes over a low heat without browning. Gradually blend in the milk and cook, stirring, over medium heat until thickened. Mix in the tuna, onion, pimento, Worcestershire sauce and salt. Cook over a low heat, stirring often, for 10 minutes. Pour the mixture into a non-stick casserole or one coated with non-stick spray. Mix the breadcrumbs and Parmesan cheese and sprinkle over the top. Bake at 375F/190C/Gas 5 for 20 minutes or until the top is browned.

Notes

CHEESE

Luncheon Lasagne

Serves 4

*145 calories
per serving*

1 lb	*eggplant*	450 g	1 lb
1 cup	*Basic Tomato Sauce (see page 154)*	225 ml	8 fl oz
1½ cups	*low-fat cottage cheese*	350 g	12 oz
¼ cup	*Parmesan cheese, grated*	25 g	1 oz

While preheating the broiler, cut the unpeeled eggplant into ¼-in/5-mm slices. Place the slices in a single layer in a pan coated with non-stick spray (or in a non-stick pan) and broil for 5 minutes; turn the slices and broil the other side for 5 minutes. Repeat with all the slices. In a casserole, layer one-third of the tomato sauce, half the eggplant slices, all the cottage cheese, the remaining eggplant slices and the remaining tomato sauce. Sprinkle the Parmesan cheese over the top. Bake about 25 minutes, until bubbly, at 375F/190C/Gas 5.

Three-Cheese Quiche

9 in	*pastry crust, unbaked*	23 cm	9 in
½ cup	*button mushrooms, sliced*	40 g	1½ oz
¾ cup	*Cheddar cheese, grated*	75 g	3 oz
3	*eggs*	3	3
½ cup	*skim milk*	125 ml	4 fl oz
1 cup	*low-fat cottage cheese*	225 g	8 oz
1½ tsp	*cornstarch*	1½ tsp	1½ tsp
½ tsp	*dried dill weed*	½ tsp	½ tsp
½ tsp	*mustard powder*	½ tsp	½ tsp
2 tbls	*Parmesan cheese*	2 tbls	2 tbls

Bake the crust at 425F/220C/Gas 7 for 10 minutes or until the edges are lightly browned. Remove the crust from the oven and reduce the heat to 350F/180C/Gas 4. Spread the mushrooms and Cheddar cheese evenly over the bottom of the crust. In a blender, mix together the eggs, milk, cottage cheese, cornstarch, dill weed and mustard powder at low speed until well blended. Carefully pour the mixture into the crust and sprinkle with the Parmesan cheese. Bake for 35 to 45 minutes, until a knife can be inserted just off center and withdrawn cleanly.

* This quiche can be served immediately, piping hot, or can be eaten cold. It reheats well too.

* Cut the calories to 245 per serving by using reduced-calorie cheese instead of ordinary Cheddar.

Macaroni and Cheese Casserole

Serves 6   *125 calories*
                                                                       per serving

1⅓ cups	uncooked macaroni	150 g	5 oz
1⅔ cups	button mushrooms, sliced	125 g	4 oz
1¾ cups	onion, finely chopped	225 g	8 oz
⅓ cup	green pepper, seeded, cored, chopped	50 g	2 oz
1 cup	Cheddar cheese, coarsely grated	125 g	4 oz
¼ tsp	black pepper	¼ tsp	¼ tsp
⅛ tsp	paprika	⅛ tsp	⅛ tsp

Cook the macaroni in boiling unsalted water for about 10 minutes, or until it is 'al dente'. Drain, rinse and drain again. Meanwhile, steam the mushrooms, onions and green pepper until just tender, about 10 minutes; stir to mix. Coat a casserole with non-stick spray. Place the drained macaroni in the dish, then layer the vegetables over, and cover with the grated cheese. Sprinkle the top with black pepper and paprika. Bake for 15 minutes at 350F/180C/Gas 4. Brown the top under the broiler for about 5 minutes.

* Serve as a side dish, instead of potatoes or rice, in the portion size suggested above. Or serve the dish in larger portions for a light luncheon or supper course.

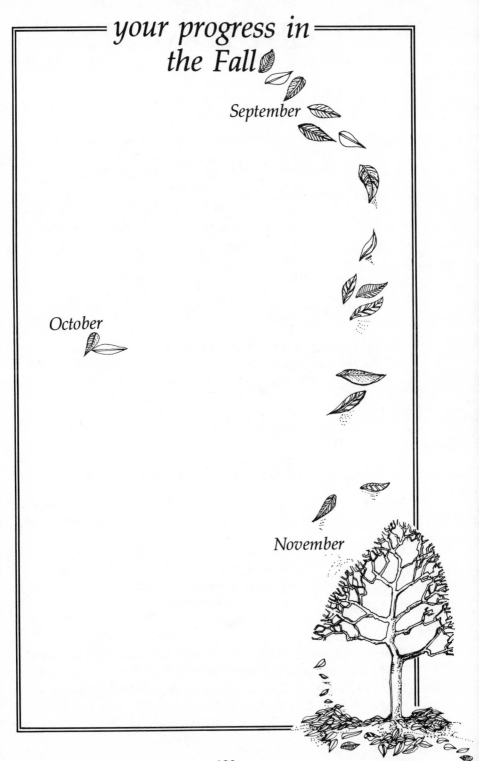

your progress in the Fall

September

October

November

LIGHT LUNCHES

Chicken Sandwich

Makes 1 sandwich   *180 calories*

1 tbls	*plain low-fat yoghurt*	1 tbls	1 tbls
1 tsp	*mustard*	1 tsp	1 tsp
2	*thin slices of bread*	2	2
2 oz	*thinly sliced chicken*	50 g	2 oz
1	*lettuce leaf*	1	1

Mix the yoghurt and mustard and spread it on the bread slices. Put the chicken and lettuce on top of one slice and cover with the other slice. Cut in quarters to serve.

French Toast

Serves 1   *170 calories per serving*

1	*egg*	1	1
¼ cup	*skim milk*	4 tbls	4 tbls
2	*thin slices of bread*	2	2
	sugar substitute equivalent to 1 tsp sugar		

Beat the egg and milk together in a shallow dish. Soak the bread in the mixture, turning once, until all the liquid is absorbed. Coat a small non-stick frying pan with non-stick spray, place over medium heat and cook the bread on both sides until brown. Sprinkle with sugar substitute and serve.

Stuffed Tomato

Serves 4

4	*medium tomatoes*	4	4
4	*egg whites, lightly beaten*	4	4
¾ cup	*tuna, canned in brine*	175 g	6 oz
4	*medium onions, finely chopped*	4	4
4	*celery stalks, finely chopped*	4	4
1 tbls	*low-calorie mayonnaise*	1 tbls	1 tbls
	pepper to taste		

Scoop out the centers of the tomatoes, taking care not to pierce the walls. Turn them upside-down to drain. Mix together all the remaining ingredients and season well with pepper. Divide the filling between the tomatoes, piling it up in a dome. Serve well chilled.

Spanish Omelet

Makes 1 omelet

1	*egg, well beaten*	1	1
¼ cup	*Basic Tomato Sauce (see page* 154)	50 ml	2 fl oz
1 oz	*low-fat Mozzarella cheese*	25 g	1 oz

Use a non-stick pan, or coat a pan with non- stick spray. Pour the egg into the pan and spread evenly. Cook well on one side. Just before folding, add cheese. Fold over and continue to cook until cheese melts. Heat tomato sauce. When the omelet is cooked, spoon the sauce over and serve at once.

Devilled Eggs

Serves 4

45 calories
per serving

2	hard-boiled eggs	2	2
1 tsp	reduced-calorie mayonnaise	1 tsp	1 tsp
1 tsp	vinegar	1 tsp	1 tsp
⅛ tsp	mustard powder	⅛ tsp	⅛ tsp
1 pinch	paprika	1 pinch	1 pinch

Cut the eggs in half lengthwise and remove the yolks. Mash the yolks with the mayonnaise, vinegar and mustard until smooth. Pipe or spoon the mixture into the egg whites and sprinkle with paprika.

Tomato Egg Bake

Serves 4

100 calories
per serving

4	medium tomatoes	4	4
	salt to taste		
	black pepper to taste		
4	eggs	4	4
1 tsp	fresh parsley, chopped	1 tsp	1 tsp
¼ cup	water	4 tbls	4 tbls

Cut a small slice from the top of each tomato and scoop out the pulp, leaving a thick tomato shell. Season the insides with salt and pepper. Break an egg into each tomato shell and sprinkle with parsley. Put the water in a baking dish just large enough to hold the tomatoes. Place the tomatoes in the dish and bake at 400F/200C/Gas 6 for about 5 minutes or until the eggs are cooked to desired firmness. Serve immediately.

Tuna Sandwich

Makes 1 sandwich   *180 calories*

2 oz	canned tuna in brine, drained	50 g	2 oz
1	small celery stick, finely chopped	1	1
2	green onions, finely chopped	2	2
2 tbls	plain low-fat yoghurt	2 tbls	2 tbls
1 tsp	mild mustard	1 tsp	1 tsp
2	thin slices of bread	2	2

Mix the tuna with the celery, green onion, yoghurt and mustard. Spread on one slice of bread, cover with the second slice and cut the sandwich in quarters to serve.

3 Egg-white Omelet

Serves 1   *115 calories*

1 tsp	margarine	7 g	¼ oz
¼ cup	green pepper, seeded, cored, chopped	40 g	1½ oz
¼ cup	onions, chopped	40 g	1½ oz
½ cup	button mushrooms, sliced	25 g	1 oz
3	egg whites	3	3

Melt the margarine in a small frying pan. Add the pepper, onion and mushrooms and cook gently for about 10 minutes until the onions and peppers are tender. Remove from the pan and keep hot. Coat the pan with non-stick spray, if necessary, and put the pan over medium heat. Beat the egg whites just until they are runny. When the pan is hot, pour in the eggs, tilting the pan to let the eggs coat the base. Cook until firm, lifting the edges to allow the liquid egg to run underneath. Remove from the heat and spoon the hot vegetables over one half of the omelet. Fold the omelet over and slide it on to a serving plate.

VEGETABLES

Italian Baked Tomatoes

Serves 4

*115 calories
per serving*

2 tbls	*margarine*	25 g	1 oz
¼ cup	*dried breadcrumbs*	25 g	1 oz
2 tbls	*Parmesan cheese, grated*	2 tbls	2 tbls
1 tsp	*garlic powder*	1 tsp	1 tsp
4	*medium tomatoes*	4	4
3 tbls	*low-calorie mayonnaise*	3 tbls	3 tbls

Melt the margarine and add the breadcrumbs, cheese and garlic powder. Stir well. Halve the tomatoes and place, cut side up, in a baking dish that has been coated with non-stick spray. Spread the mayonnaise evenly on each tomato half, then spoon the breadcrumb mixture on top. Bake for 15 to 20 minutes, until just tender, at 350F/180C/Gas 4.

Baked Spinach

Serves 4

*132 calories
per serving*

2 tbls	*margarine*	25 g	1 oz
¼ cup	*onion, chopped*	40 g	1½ oz
2 cups	*frozen spinach-thawed, drained, chopped*	200 g	14 oz
½ cup	*skim milk*	125 ml	4 fl oz
2	*eggs, well beaten*	2	2

Melt the margarine in a frying pan and sauté the onions. Add the drained spinach and mix well. Heat the mixture through, then remove it from the heat and add the milk and beaten egg. Put the mixture into a non-stick pan, or small casserole that has been coated with non-stick spray. Bake for 30 minutes at 350F/180C/Gas 4.

Stir-Fry Vegetables

Serves 4

about 45 calories
per serving

2 tsp	*vegetable oil*	2 tsp	2 tsp
4 cups	*any low-calorie vegetables, sliced*	575 g	1¼ lb

Heat the oil in a large frying pan or wok. Add the vegetables and stir-fry over a medium-high heat until they are tender but still crisp, about 3 minutes.

*For extra flavor and fragrance, add a slice of fresh ginger and/ or a lightly crushed garlic clove to the oil while heating it. Remove it before adding the vegetables.
*They may be served with Sweet and Sour Sauce (see page 157), adding 25 calories per serving.

Cheese Whipped Potatoes

Serves 4

105 calories
per serving

1 lb	*potatoes, peeled and quartered*	450 g	1 lb
¼ cup	*low-fat cottage cheese*	50 g	2 oz
¼ cup	*skim milk*	4 tbls	4 tbls
to taste	*white pepper*	to taste	to taste
1 tbls	*Parmesan cheese, grated*	1 tbls	1 tbls
1 tbls	*margarine, melted*	1 tbls	1 tbls
to taste	*fresh chives, snipped*	to taste	to taste

Boil the potatoes in unsalted water until fork-tender, about 20 minutes. Drain well, making sure the potatoes are completely dry. Mash the potatoes by hand, then put them into an electric mixer and set aside. In a blender purée cottage cheese and milk until smooth. Add the mixture to the potatoes and whip them together until fluffy. Season with white pepper. Transfer the whipped potatoes to a shallow baking pan and smooth the top. Sprinkle it evenly with the Parmesan cheese, then drizzle with the melted margarine. Brown under the broiler until the top is golden. Garnish with the snipped chives.

Broccoli Soufflé

Serves 4

95 calories
per serving

2 cups	broccoli, finely chopped	200 g	7 oz
½ cup	onion, chopped	75 g	3 oz
2	egg whites	2	2
⅓ cup	mozzarella cheese, grated	40 g	1½ oz
½ cup	low-fat cottage cheese	125 g	4 oz
1 pinch	paprika	1 pinch	1 pinch

Steam the broccoli and onion together (or cook in a small amount of boiling water) until just tender; drain well. Meanwhile, whisk the egg whites until they form stiff peaks. Put the drained vegetables into a casserole. Mix the mozzarella cheese into the hot vegetables, then blend in the cottage cheese. Gently fold in the whisked egg whites. Sprinkle the top with paprika. Bake for 30 minutes at 350F/180C/Gas 4.

Indian Rice

Serves 4

130 calories
per serving

⅔ cup	brown rice	125 g	4½ oz
¼ cup	onion, chopped	40 g	1½ oz
⅓ cup	canned or fresh tomato, chopped	75 g	2½ oz
¼ cup	green pepper, seeded, cored, chopped	40 g	1½ oz
1 tsp	curry powder	1 tsp	1 tsp
2 tsp	margarine, salted	7 g	¼ oz
1⅓ cups	unsalted chicken stock	325 ml	11 fl oz

Coat a casserole with non-stick spray. Put all the ingredients in a bowl and stir well to mix. Transfer to the casserole, cover and bake for 1 hour at 350F/180C/Gas 4.

Herbed Carrots

Serves 4

30 calories
per serving*

¼ cup	*water*	4 tbls	4 tbls
2 tbls	*lemon juice*	2 tbls	2 tbls
1 tbls	*margarine*	15 g	½ oz
¼ tsp	*ground allspice*	¼ tsp	¼ tsp
2½ cups	*carrots, sliced diagonally*	350 g	12 oz
2 tbls	*fresh parsley, finely chopped*	2 tbls	2 tbls

In a saucepan, combine the water, lemon juice, margarine and allspice. Bring to the boil, stirring occasionally. Add the carrots, bring back to the boil, then reduce the heat to medium low. Cook gently for 5 to 8 minutes, stirring occasionally to coat the carrots. (The thickness of the carrot slices will determine the cooking time.) When cooked, the carrots should be covered in a thin glaze, with no water remaining in the pan. Toss with the parsley and serve.

Pineapple Acorn Squash

Serves 4

*75 calories
per serving*

1 (1¼ lb)	*acorn squash*	1 (575 g)	1 (1¼lb)
1 cup	*crushed pineapple, canned in own juice*	275 g	10 oz
1 pinch	*ground cinnamon*	1 pinch	1 pinch

Halve the squash and remove the seeds. Place each half, cut side down, in a pan coated with non-stick spray. Bake for 40 minutes at 350F/180C/Gas 4. Turn the squash cut side up, divide the pineapple between the two halves and sprinkle with cinnamon. Continue baking for a further 20 minutes. Cut each piece in half before serving.

Cabbage in the Oven

Serves 4

*165 calories
per serving*

3 cups	cabbage, finely shredded	300 g	11 oz
1½ cups	canned tomatoes, unsalted	350 g	12 oz
1 pinch	salt	1 pinch	1 pinch
1 pinch	paprika	1 pinch	1 pinch
½ cup	Cheddar cheese, grated	50 g	2 oz
½ cup	dried breadcrumbs	50 g	2 oz
1 tbls	margarine	15 g	½ oz

Steam the cabbage for 5 minutes; drain well. Combine the tomatoes, salt and paprika in a saucepan and simmer for 15 minutes, stirring occasionally. Coat a casserole with non-stick spray. Place alternate layers of tomato and cabbage in the casserole, starting with the tomato. Sprinkle the top with the grated cheese and breadcrumbs and dot with margarine. Bake uncovered for 30 minutes at 325F/160C/Gas 3.

Curried Mushrooms

Serves 4

*120 calories
per serving*

2 lb	fresh mushrooms, sliced	900 g	2 lb
¼ cup	onion, chopped	40 g	1½ oz
1 tbls	vegetable oil	1 tbls	1 tbls
10 oz	can of condensed chicken soup	275 g	10 oz
to taste	curry powder	to taste	to taste

In a large frying pan, fry the mushrooms and onions in the oil until soft. Meanwhile, in a large bowl, combine the soup, half a soup can of water and curry powder to taste. Mix well until smooth, then add the mushroom mixture to the bowl and stir well. Transfer to a casserole that has been coated with non-stick spray. Cover and bake for 45 minutes at 350F/180C/Gas 4.

Artichokes with Herby Sauce

Serves 4   *about 95 calories*
                                                      per serving

4	*medium artichokes*	4	4
1 tbls	*vinegar*	1 tbls	1 tbls
3 cups	*water*	700 ml	¼ pt
¼ cup	*lemon juice*	4 tbls	4 tbls
½ cup	*onion, chopped*	75 g	3 oz
1	*celery sticks (with leaves)*	4	4
1	*bay leaf*	1	1

Sauce

½ cup	*plain yoghurt*	125 ml	4 fl oz
½ cup	*hot broth (reserved from cooking water)*	125 ml	4 fl oz
2-4	*garlic cloves, minced*	2-4	2-4
½ tsp	*basil*	½ tsp	½ tsp
¼ tsp	*thyme*	¼ tsp	¼ tsp
⅛ tsp	*white pepper*	⅛ tsp	⅛ tsp

Prepare the artichokes one by one. Bend the stem at the base until it snaps off, then trim the base so the artichoke can stand upright. Break off the small leaves at the base. Lay the artichoke on its side and cut ¾ in/2 cm off the top of the center cone of leaves. With the scissors trim off the sharp points on the rest of the leaves. Rinse well under cold running water. To minimize discoloration, drop it into a large bowl of cold water containing 1 tbls of vinegar per 5 cups/1.1 litre/2 pt water until all the artichokes are prepared.

Put the water, lemon juice, onion, celery sticks and bay leaf in a large saucepan. Either stand the artichokes upright directly in the water, or place them in a steamer, stem side up. Bring the liquid to a boil, then reduce to a simmer. Cover and cook about 45 minutes, or until you can readily pluck a leaf. Reserving the cooking broth, drain the artichokes upside down while you make the sauce. Strain the cooking broth and measure out ½ cup/125 ml/4 fl oz.

To make the sauce, put the yoghurt into a small pan, stir in the cornstarch and gradually pour on the stock, stirring all the time. Add the other ingredients, bring to the boil, leave to infuse for a few minutes. Stir again, then divide into 4 small containers and serve alongside the artichokes.

* By going 'sauceless' you can cut back the calories by 25.

Stuffed Baked Potatoes

Serves 4

90 calories
per serving

2 (5½ oz each)	potatoes	2(150 g each)	2 (5½oz each)
1 cup	low-fat cottage cheese	225 g	8 oz
2 tsp	dried chives	2 tsp	2 tsp
1 pinch	garlic powder	1 pinch	1 pinch

Scrub the potatoes well, pierce them with a fork and bake at 400F/200C/Gas 6 until fully cooked, about 40 minutes. Cut the baked potatoes in half and scoop the flesh into a bowl. Place the potato shells in a baking pan and return them to the oven. Mash together the cottage cheese and potato. Mix in the chives and garlic powder. Divide the potato mixture into the potato shells. Return the filled potatoes to the oven for 5 to 10 minutes, until heated through.

Rice Pilaff

Serves 4

100 calories
per serving

⅔ cup	brown rice	125 g	4½ oz
¼ cup	onion, chopped	40 g	1½ oz
1⅓ cups	unsalted chicken stock	325 ml	11 fl oz

Coat a casserole with non-stick spray and put the rice, onions and stock into it. Stir to mix, cover and bake for 1 hour at 350F/180C/Gas 4.

*You can make as much Rice Pilaff as you want - just remember to use twice as much liquid as rice and increase the onion accordingly. It's easy and delicious, and a good company dish.

*Green onions look nice in this. Be sure to include the tops.

*For convenience you may wish to use canned bouillon, diluted as directed.

Ratatouille

Serves 4

160 calories
per serving

1 cup	onions, chopped	175 g	6 oz
¼ cup	olive oil	4 tbls	4 tbls
1 lb	eggplant, peeled and diced	450 g	1 lb
1½ cups	green pepper-seeded, cored, chopped	250 g	9 oz
3	medium tomatoes, chopped	3	3
1 lb	zucchini, sliced	450 g	1 lb
⅔	celery, chopped	75 g	3 oz
1	garlic clove, mashed	1	1
1 tsp	dried basil	1 tsp	1 tsp
1 tsp	mixed dried herbs	1 tsp	1 tsp
1 pinch	dried oregano	1 pinch	1 pinch
to taste	black pepper	to taste	to taste

Sauté the onions in the oil until soft. Add the eggplant and peppers and cook for another 5 minutes. Add the tomatoes, zucchini and celery and simmer, covered, for about 45 minutes. Add the garlic and herbs during the last 5 minutes of cooking. Serve hot or cold.

Steamed Bulgar

Serves 4

100 calories
per serving

2 cups	unsalted chicken stock	475 ml	16 fl oz
1 cup	bulgar	150 g	5½ oz

Bring the stock to the boil. Add the bulgar and reduce the heat. Simmer for 20 minutes, or until all the liquid is absorbed.

Stuffed Mushrooms

Serves 4

110 calories per serving

16	large fresh mushrooms	16	16
1 tbls	margarine	15 g	½ oz
3	green onions, finely chopped	3	3
1 tbls	fresh parsley, chopped	1 tbls	1 tbls
¼ cup	dried breadcrumbs	25 g	1 oz
3 tbls	Parmesan cheese, grated	3 tbls	3 tbls

Pull out the mushroom stems and chop them. Melt the margarine in a non-stick pan. Stir in the chopped mushroom stems, green onions, parsley and breadcrumbs. Cook over a low heat for about 15 minutes, stirring occasionally. Fill each mushroom cap with a little of the stuffing and place them in a non-stick baking pan. Sprinkle with the Parmesan cheese and bake for 15 minutes at 350F/180C/Gas 4. Serve immediately.

Zucchini Pomodoro

Serves 4

40 calories per serving

2 lb	zucchini or summer squash	900 g	2 lb
¾ cup	Basic Tomato Sauce (see page 154)	175 ml	6 fl oz

Steam the zucchini or squash until just tender; drain well. Mix the vegetable thoroughly into the sauce and pour the mixture into a baking dish. Bake until browned on top, about 30 minutes, at 400F/200C/Gas 6.
*Instead of zucchini or summer squash, you can substitute the same amount of eggplant, peeled and diced.
*For extra flavor, add ½ cup/75 g/3 oz chopped onion to the main vegetable; steam and bake as above. Calories increase by about 10 per serving.

Tomatoes in the Oven

Serves 4

*117 calories
per serving*

2 tbls	*margarine*	25 g	1 oz
¼ cup	*dried breadcrumbs*	25 g	1 oz
2 tbls	*Parmesan cheese*	2 tbls	2 tbls
1 tsp	*garlic powder*	1 tsp	1 tsp
4	*medium tomatoes*	4	4
3 tbls	*low-calorie mayonnaise*	3 tbls	3 tbls

Combine the margarine, breadcrumbs, cheese and garlic powder. Stir well. Halve the tomatoes and place them cut side up in a non-stick baking dish. Spread the mayonnaise evenly on each tomato half, then spoon the breadcrumb mixture over. Bake for 15 to 20 minutes until just tender at 350F/180C/ Gas 4.

Zucchini Casserole

Serves 4

*185 calories
per serving*

2 lb	*zucchini, sliced*	900 g	2 lb
¼ cup	*onion, chopped*	40 g	1½ oz
1	*egg*	1	1
½ cup	*skim milk*	125 ml	4 fl oz
4 oz	*low-fat milk powder*	125 g	4 oz
½ cup	*mozzarella cheese, grated*	50 g	2 oz
¼ cup	*Parmesan cheese, grated*	25 g	1 oz

Put the zucchini and onions in a non-stick frying pan and fry them, using no fat, until the zucchini is limp and the onions partially cooked. Put the egg, skim milk and powdered milk into a casserole and beat until well mixed. Add the zucchini, onion mixture, and half the mozzarella cheese and stir to mix. Sprinkle the Parmesan cheese on top. Cover and bake for 45 minutes at 350F/180C/Gas 4.

SAUCES

Basic Tomato Sauce

Makes 1 qt/950 ml/32 fl oz

*25 calories
per ¼ cup/60 ml/2 fl oz*

3 lb	tomatoes, canned, unsalted, with juice	1.4 kg	3 lb
1 cup	onions, chopped	175 g	6 oz
1 cup	green pepper, seeded, cored, chopped	175 g	6 oz
1 tsp	dried oregano	1 tsp	1 tsp
½ tsp	dried basil	½ tsp	½ tsp
½ tsp	black pepper	½ tsp	½ tsp
½ tsp	garlic powder	½ tsp	½ tsp

In a large pan combine the chopped vegetables, herbs and garlic powder. Simmer gently, stirring occasionally, for about 2 hours until reduced and thickened. Measure the sauce and make up to 1 qt/950 ml/32 fl oz with water.
* To make a smooth sauce, purée the ingredients together in a blender after cooking.
* For convenience, you can freeze the sauce in ice cube trays, then turn out and transfer to a freezer bag and store until needed.

Imitation Sour Cream

Makes 1½ cups/350 ml/12 fl oz

*30 calories
per serving (2 tbls)*

1½ cups	low-fat cottage cheese	350 g	12 oz
1 tsp	lemon juice	1 tsp	1 tsp

Put the cheese and lemon juice into a blender and blend for 1 minute, until smooth and creamy. Store in a covered container in the refrigerator.

Barbecue Sauce

Makes 3 cups/700 ml/24 fl oz

*5 calories
per tablespoon*

12 oz	tomato paste (unsalted)	350 g	12 oz
4½ cups	water	1 litre	1¾ pt
½ cup	vinegar	125 ml	4 fl oz
¼	lemon juice	4 tbls	4 tbls
	sugar substitute equivalent to 2 tbls sugar		
¼ cup	onion, finely chopped	40 g	1½ oz
1 tbls	garlic powder	1 tbls	1 tbls
1 tbls	onion powder	1 tbls	1 tbls
2 tsp	mustard powder	2 tsp	2 tsp
½ tsp	paprika	½ tsp	½ tsp
⅛ tsp	allspice	⅛ tsp	⅛ tsp
⅛ tsp	cinnamon	⅛ tsp	⅛ tsp
1 pinch	ground cloves	1 pinch	1 pinch

Put the tomato paste into a large pan and blend in the remaining ingredients. Bring to the boil, then lower the heat and simmer, stirring occasionally, for up to 2 hours until the sauce has thickened.

Low-Calorie French Dressing

Makes ¾ cup/175 ml/6 fl oz

*8 calories
per serving (2 tbls)*

½ cup	tomato juice	125 ml	4 fl oz
2 tbls	lemon juice or cider vinegar	2 tbls	2 tbls
1 tbls	onion, finely chopped	1 tbls	1 tbls
1 tbls	green pepper, finely chopped	1 tbls	1 tbls
⅛ tsp	black pepper	⅛ tsp	⅛ tsp

Combine all the ingredients in a jar. Cover and shake well.

Quick Tomato Sauce

Makes 1 cup/225 ml/8 fl oz　　　　　　　　　　　*25 calories*
per ¼ cup/50 ml/2 fl oz

2	medium tomatoes, chopped	2	2
¼ cup	water	4 tbls	4 tbls
¼ cup	onion, finely chopped	40 g	1½ oz
¼ cup	green pepper, seeded, cored, chopped	40 g	1½ oz
¼ tsp	dried oregano	¼ tsp	¼ tsp
¼ tsp	dried basil, thyme or marjoram	¼ tsp	¼ tsp
⅛ tsp	black pepper	⅛ tsp	⅛ tsp
	garlic powder to taste		

Purée the tomatoes with the water in a blender. Pour the purée into a saucepan and stir in the remaining ingredients. Cook over a low heat, stirring occasionally, for 15 minutes.

Spanish Sauce

Makes 2 cups/475 ml/16 fl oz　　　　　　　　　　*25 calories*
per ½ cup/125 ml/4 fl oz

¼ cup	onion, finely chopped	40 g	1½ oz
¼ cup	green pepper, seeded, cored, chopped	40 g	1½ oz
⅓ cup	water	5 tbls	5 tbls
1 cup	canned tomatoes, unsalted, drained, chopped	225 g	8 oz
¼ cup	tomato juice (reserved from can)	4 tbls	4 tbls
¼ cup	canned mushrooms, rinsed, chopped	50 g	2 oz

Cook the onion and green pepper in the water until soft. Add the tomatoes, the reserved juice and the mushrooms. Simmer, partially covered, for 15 minutes, until the sauce has thickened. If necessary, add more juice from the can to make up the total volume.

Sweet and Sour Sauce

Makes ⅔ cup/150 ml/5 fl oz

*15 calories
per tablespoon*

4 tsp	cornstarch	4 tsp	4 tsp
	brown sugar substitute equivalent to		
	2 tsp sugar		
½ cup	pineapple juice	125 ml	4 fl oz
2 tbls	vinegar	2 tbls	2 tbls
¼ tsp	black pepper	¼ tsp	¼ tsp
¼ tsp	ground ginger	¼ tsp	¼ tsp

Stir the cornstarch and sugar substitute into half the pineapple juice and blend well, then add the remaining juice along with the vinegar, pepper and ginger. Slowly bring to a boil, stirring, then lower the heat and cook for about 1 minute, until thickened.

* To make a simple Chinese stir-fry sauce, blend 4 tsp cornstarch with ¼ cup/60 ml/2 fl oz unsalted stock, then stir in a further ¾ cup/175 ml/6 fl oz stock. Cook as above.

Cranberry and Orange Relish

Makes 4 cups/900 ml/1½ pints

*5 calories
per serving (2 tbls)*

1 lb	fresh or frozen cranberries	450 g	1 lb
2	small oranges, segmented, seeded	2	2
2 tbls	grated orange rind	2 tbls	2 tbls
	sugar substitute equivalent to		
	1 cup/225 g/8 oz sugar		

Place all the ingredients in a blender. Blend until the mixture is coarse and grainy. Store in a covered container in the refrigerator for 2-3 days before using.

Mushroom Sauce

Makes 1 cup/225 ml/8 fl oz   *75 calories*
per ¼ cup/60 ml/2 fl oz

2 tsp	cornstarch	2 tsp	2 tsp
¾ cup	skim milk	175 ml	6 fl oz
2 tsp	oil or melted margarine	2 tsp	2 tsp
¾ cup	Mozzarella cheese, shredded	40 g	1½ oz
¼ cup	canned mushroom pieces, drained	50 g	2 oz

Stir the cornstarch into the cold milk and blend well. Stir the oil or melted margarine into the milk. Slowly bring to a boil, stirring, then lower the heat and cook for about 1 minute until thickened. Remove from the heat, add the cheese and stir until melted and smooth. Add the mushrooms. Use as a sauce for casseroles.

Orange Sauce

Makes ½ cup/125 ml/4 fl oz   *10 calories*
per tablespoon

1½ tsp	cornstarch	1½ tsp	1½ tsp
½ cup	orange juice	125 ml	4 fl oz
2 tsp	orange peel, grated	2 tsp	2 tsp
	sugar substitute equivalent to 1 tbls sugar		

In a small saucepan, blend the cornstarch with the orange juice, then stir in the orange peel and sugar substitute (if using). Slowly bring to the boil, then simmer for a few minutes until the sauce is clear and slightly thickened. Serve over baked chicken.
* For a spicier sauce, good with pork, add ¼ tsp cinnamon and 4 whole cloves. Remove the cloves before serving.

your progress in Winter

December

January

February

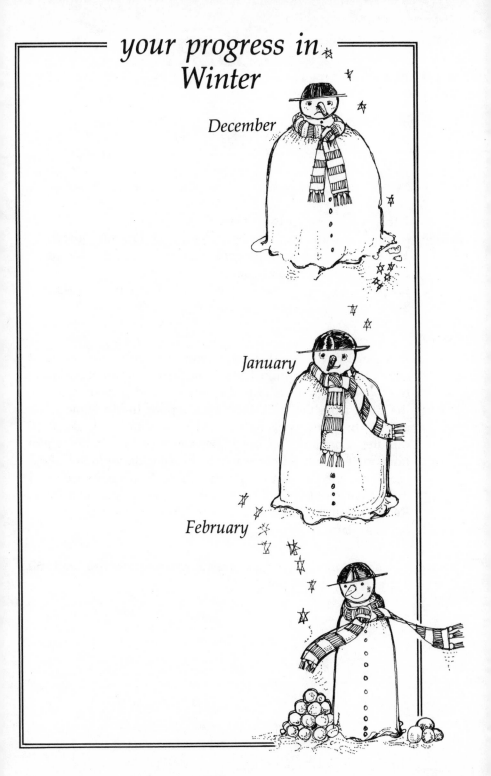

DESSERTS

Apple Chill

Serves 4

*55 calories
per serving*

1 tbls	powdered gelatin	1 tbls	1 tbls
½ cup	water	125 ml	4 fl oz
1 cup	unsweetened apple juice	225 ml	8 fl oz
2	small apples	2	2
1 tsp	lemon juice	1 tsp	1 tsp
8	seedless grapes	8	8

In a small bowl, sprinkle the gelatin over the water and let it soften for about 5 minutes. Stand the bowl in a pan of hot water over low heat and stir until the gelatin has dissolved. Remove the bowl from the heat, then slowly pour in the apple juice, stirring to blend well. Refrigerate until almost set, about 30 minutes. Core and dice the apples and toss them in the lemon juice mixed with a little water to prevent discoloration. Fold them into the partially set gelatin. Place 2 grapes in each of 4 individual molds and then divide the gelatin between them. Refrigerate until firm, about 4 hours. Just before serving unmold on to 4 plates.

* To add more color to this refreshing dessert, choose 1 red and 1 green or yellow apple.

Tropical Delight

Serves 4

40 calories per serving

1½ tsp	*powdered gelatin*	1½ tsp	1½ tsp
¼ cup	*cold water*	4 tbls	4 tbls
	sugar substitute equivalent to 2 tsp sugar		
3 tbls	*pineapple juice concentrate, thawed*	3 tbls	3 tbls
¾ tsp	*rum flavoring*	¾ tsp	¾ tsp
½ tsp	*coconut flavoring*	½ tsp	½ tsp
¼ cup	*evaporated skim milk, well chilled*	4 tbls	4 tbls
¼ cup	*crushed pineapple canned in juice, drained*	65 g	2½ oz

In a small bowl, sprinkle the gelatin over the water and let it soften for 5 minutes. Stand the bowl in a pan of hot water over low heat and stir until the gelatin has dissolved. Remove the bowl from the heat and stir in the sugar substitute, juice concentrate and flavorings. Using a chilled bowl and beaters, beat the milk until stiff peaks form. Add the gelatin mixture and beat again until thick and creamy. Fold in the crushed pineapple. Pour into a freezerproof container, cover and freeze at least 1 hour.

* Make sure the evaporated milk is well chilled, otherwise it cannot be successfully whipped. Store it in the coldest part of the refrigerator for at last 12 hours.

* Other frozen juice concentrates may be substituted for pineapple.

Dessert Omelet

Serves 1

160 calories
per serving

3	egg whites	3	3
¼ cup	low-fat cottage cheese	50 g	2 oz
	brown sugar substitute equivalent to 2 tbls sugar		
¼ cup	banana, sliced	50 g	2 oz
¼ cup	strawberries, sliced	50 g	2 oz

Use a small, non-stick frying pan or coat a pan with non-stick spray and put it over medium heat. Beat the egg whites just until they are runny. When the pan is hot, pour in the eggs, tilting the pan to let the eggs coat the base. Cook until firm, lifting the edges to let liquid egg run underneath. Remove from the heat and spoon the cottage cheese on to one half of the omelet. Fold it in half and slide the omelet on to a plate. Sprinkle the sugar substitute on the omelet, then top with the banana and strawberries.

Strawberry Banana Chantilly

Serves 4

85 calories
per serving

1½ cups	strawberries	225 g	8 oz
2	bananas	2	2
½ cup	vanilla yoghurt	125 ml	4 fl oz

Cut the strawberries in half; reserve 4 halves for decoration and divide the remaining between 4 serving bowls. Cut the bananas in half lengthwise and slice them. Divide the bananas between the bowls, gently mixing them with the strawberries. Spoon the vanilla yoghurt on top, decorate with a reserved strawberry half and serve at once.

Prune and Orange Cake

Makes 12 slices

*115 calories
per slice*

¼ cup	margarine, softened	50 g	2 oz
½ cup	instant non-fat milk, powdered	50 g	2 oz
1	egg	1	1
¾ cup	orange juice	175 ml	6 fl oz
1 cup	wholewheat flour	165 g	5½ oz
1½ tsp	baking powder	1½ tsp	1½ tsp
½ tsp	salt	½ tsp	½ tsp
8	prunes, pitted and finely chopped	8	8
1 tbls	orange rind, grated	1 tbls	1 tbls

Use a 9x5-in/23x13-cm non-stick loaf pan, or coat one with non-stick spray. Cream the margarine and slowly add the powdered milk, beating until light and creamy. Beat in the egg and orange juice. In a separate bowl, mix the flour, baking powder and salt. Stir in the chopped prunes and orange rind. Add this mixture to the orange juice mixture and blend together well. Pour into the loaf pan and bake for 45 minutes at 325F/160C/Gas 3 or until firm to the touch. Leave in the pan for 5 minutes, then turn out on to a rack to cool.

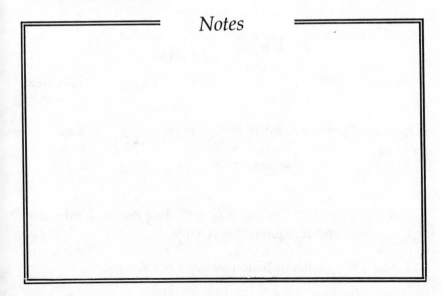

Notes

Baked Apples

Serves 4

40 calories
per serving

2	medium apples	2	2
½tsp	lemon juice	½ tsp	½ tsp
½ tsp	ground cinnamon	½ tsp	½ tsp
	brown sugar substitute equivalent to 2 tsp sugar		
1 cup	diet soft drink	225 ml	8 fl oz

Cut the apples in half and remove the cores. Coat the flesh with the lemon juice and place the apples, cut side up, in a small baking dish. Stir the cinnamon and sugar substitute into the soft drink and pour it over the apples. Bake for about 30 minutes at 350F/180C/Gas 4 or until the apples are quite soft when pierced with a fork. During cooking, baste them once or twice with the liquid. Serve warm or cold.

* Ginger ale is a good choice, as it subtly adds to the spiciness. You could also use a fruit-flavored soft drink such as lemon or orange.

Fruit Salad

Serves 4

76 calories
per serving

½ cup	pineapple chunks, canned, in juice	75 g	3 oz
1 cup	bananas, sliced	175 g	6 oz
½ cup	seedless grapes	50 g	2 oz

Mix all the ingredients together, including the juice from the can. Cover and refrigerate. Serve chilled.

* Add 1 tsp vanilla or lemon yoghurt per serving.

Strawberry Meringue Pie

Serves 4

80 calories per serving

2	egg whites	2	2
	sugar substitute equivalent to ½ cup/4 oz sugar		
½ tsp	vanilla extract	½ tsp	½ tsp
½ tsp	lemon peel	½ tsp	½ tsp
1½ cups	strawberries	225 g	8 oz
¼ tsp	vanilla yoghurt	4 tsp	4 tsp

Beat the eggs until stiff peaks form. Add the sugar substitute a little at a time, beating well after each addition. Fold in the vanilla extract and lemon peel. Spread the meringue evenly on a non-stick pie pan, making sure to coat the sides. Bake for 1 hour at 250F/130C/Gas ½ until dry. Just before serving, mash the strawberries, reserving 4 for decoration. Spoon the strawberry purée into the meringue shell. Serve the pie with 1 tsp yoghurt and a whole strawberry on top of each slice.

* The meringue can also be shaped into a nest; draw an 8-in/20-cm circle on a piece of non-stick silicone paper and line a cookie sheet with the paper. Spread the meringue within the circle, heaping it at the sides to form a nest.

Baked Custard

Serves 4

85 calories per serving

2	*eggs*	2	2
2 cups	*skim milk*	475 ml	16 fl oz
	sugar substitute equivalent to 2 tsp sugar		
1 tsp	*vanilla extract*	1 tsp	1 tsp
½ tsp	*grated nutmeg*	½ tsp	½ tsp

Coat 4 custard cups or ramekins with non-stick spray. Beat the eggs, milk, sugar substitute and vanilla extract until blended. Pour into the dishes and sprinkle with nutmeg. Set the dishes in a pan filled with 1 in/25 mm water and bake for 1 hour at 325F/ 160C/Gas 3 or until a knife inserted in the center comes out clean.

Orange Freeze

Serves 4

60 calories per serving

⅝ cup	*evaporated skim milk, well chilled*	150 ml	5 fl oz
5 tbls	*frozen orange juice concentrate, thawed*	5 tbls	5 tbls
½ tsp	*vanilla extract*	½ tsp	½ tsp

Using a chilled bowl and beaters, beat the evaporated milk until stiff peaks form. Add the juice concentrate and vanilla extract and beat again until thick and creamy. Freeze until ready to serve, at least 1 hour.

* Make sure the evaporated milk is well chilled, otherwise it cannot be successfuly whipped. Store it in the coldest part of the refrigerator for at least 12 hours.

Meringue Cookies

4	egg whites	4	4
½ cup	instant non-fat milk powder	50 g	2 oz
	powdered sugar substitute		
	equivalent to ½ cup/4 oz sugar		
1 tsp	vanilla extract	1 tsp	1 tsp
1 tsp	almond extract	1 tsp	1 tsp
	cinnamon to taste		

Use a non-stick cookie sheet, coat one with non-stick spray or cover with non-stick silicone paper. Beat the egg whites until stiff peaks form. Mix the powdered milk and sugar substitute and fold into the egg whites a little at a time, beating well after each addition. Fold in the extracts. Drop by teaspoonfuls on to the cookie sheet. Bake for 1 hour at 275F/140C/Gas 1 until dry and light brown. Lightly dust each cookie with cinnamon.

Hot Pineapple with Yoghurt

8	pineapple rings, canned in juice	8	8
	brown sugar substitute equivalent to		
	1 tsp sugar		
½ cup	vanilla yoghurt	125 ml	4 fl oz

Broil the pineapple rings on one side until bubbling and starting to brown at the edges. Immediately, sprinkle over the brown sugar substitute so that it melts. Place 2 pineapple rings on each of 4 serving plates and spoon the yoghurt on top. Serve at once.

Peach Custard Pie

Serves 4

100 calories
per serving

	meringue pie crust *(see recipe on page 165)*		
1 cup	skim milk	225 ml	8 fl oz
1	egg	1	1
	sugar substitute equivalent to 2 tbls sugar		
1½ tsp	ground cinnamon	1½ tsp	1½ tsp
1 tsp	vanilla extract	1 tsp	1 tsp
2 cups	sliced peaches, canned in juice	225 g	8 oz

Heat the milk in a heavy-based saucepan until hot. Beat the egg with the sugar substitute and 1 tsp of the cinnamon. Slowly pour in the hot milk, stirring constantly until well blended. Pour back into the saucepan and cook gently, stirring with a wooden spoon, until the mixture thickens and coats the back of the spoon. Remove from the heat and add the vanilla extract. Transfer to a bowl, cover the surface of the custard with plastic wrap and refrigerate for at least 1 hour. Just before serving, spoon the custard into the meringue shell. Arrange the peach slices attractively on top. Sprinkle with the remaining ½ tsp cinnamon and serve at once.

* Use fresh peaches when in season. While the custard is chilling, slice them and toss in a little lemon juice to prevent discoloration. Refrigerate the peach slices until needed.

Cinnamon Apple Cream

Serves 4

45 calories
per serving

2 tsp	powdered gelatin	2 tsp	2 tsp
⅔ cup	water	150 ml	5 fl oz
	sugar substitute equivalent to 2½ tsp		
⅔	plain low-fat yoghurt	150 ml	5 fl oz
½ tsp	lemon juice	½ tsp	½ tsp
¼ tsp	ground cinnamon	¼ tsp	¼ tsp
⅔ cup	apple, cored, diced	65 g	2½ oz
2 tsp	seedless raisins	2 tsp	2 tsp

In a small bowl, sprinkle the gelatin over the water and let it soften for 5 minutes. Stand the bowl in a pan of hot water over low heat and stir until the gelatin has dissolved. Remove the bowl from the heat and stir in the sugar substitute. In another bowl, mix the yoghurt, lemon juice and cinnamon. Slowly add the gelatin, stirring to blend well. Refrigerate until almost set, then fold in the apple and raisins. Spoon into 4 individual molds and refrigerate until firm, about 2 hours. Just before serving, unmold on to 4 plates.

Frosty Banana

Serves 2

40 calories
per serving

Peel a well-ripened (brown speckled) banana, slice in half crosswise and tightly wrap each piece in aluminium foil. Freeze until firm, about 4 hours. Serve within 5 minutes of removing from the freezer.

BEVERAGES

Lemonade

Serves 1   *5 calories*

1 tbls	*lemon juice*	1 tbls	1 tbls
1 cup	*chilled water*	225 ml	8 fl oz
	sugar substitute equivalent to		
	2 tsp sugar		
1	*sliced lemon*	1	1
1	*sprig of mint*	1	1

Stir the ingredients together. Serve over ice cubes and decorate the glass with the lemon slice and mint sprig.

Eggnog

Serves 4   *175 calories*
                                                        per serving

4	*eggs, at room temperature*	4	4
1 qt	*skim milk*	950 ml	32 fl oz
	sugar substitute equivalent to		
	2 tsp sugar		
1 tsp	*vanilla extract*	1 tsp	1 tsp
½ tsp	*rum extract*	½ tsp	½ tsp
4	*ice cubes*	4	4
1 pinch	*nutmeg*	1 pinch	1 pinch

Immerse the eggs in boiling water for just 30 seconds, then break them into a blender. Add the milk, sugar substitute, vanilla and rum extracts and ice cubes. Blend until the ice cubes are pulverized. Pour into glasses and sprinkle each serving with nutmeg.

Hot Spiced Apple Tea

Serves 1   15 calories

1	tea bag	1	1
1 cup	boiling water	225 ml	8 fl oz
2 tbls	apple juice (unsweetened)	2 tbls	2 tbls
	sugar substitute equivalent to		
	1 tsp sugar		
½ tsp	lemon juice	½ tsp	½ tsp
¼ tsp	orange peel, grated	¼ tsp	¼ tsp
¼ tsp	cinnamon	¼ tsp	¼ tsp
1 pinch	ground cloves	1 pinch	1 pinch
1	cinnamon stick or slice of orange	1	1

Steep the tea bag in the boiling water for 3 minutes. Discard the bag and stir in the apple juice, sugar substitute, lemon juice, orange peel and spices. Serve with a cinnamon stick or orange slice.

Hot Cocoa

Serves 1   80 calories

1 tbls	cocoa	1 tbls	1 tbls
	sugar substitute equivalent to		
	1 tbls sugar		
1½ tbls	cold water	1½ tbls	1½ tbls
1 cup	skim milk	225 ml	8 fl oz
few drops	vanilla extract	few drops	few drops

In a saucepan, blend the cocoa, sugar substitute and water until smooth. Slowly bring to the boil, stirring constantly, and boil for 1 minute. Pour in the milk and heat until very hot but not boiling. Stir in the vanilla extract. Beat the hot cocoa until frothy, then serve.

Hot Spiced Tea

Serves 1   *10 calories*

1	tea bag	1	1
¼ tsp	cinnamon	¼ tsp	¼ tsp
1 pinch	ground ginger	1 pinch	1 pinch
1	whole clove	1	1
¾ cup	boiling water	175 ml	6 fl oz
4 tsp	orange juice	4 tsp	4 tsp
	sugar substitute (optional)		
	equivalent to ½ tsp sugar		
1	slice of orange or lemon	1	1

Steep the tea bag and spices in the boiling water for 3 minutes. Stir in the orange juice and sugar substitute (if used). Remove the tea bag, add the orange or lemon slice and serve.

Hot Cranberry Tea

Serves 1   *10 calories*

1	tea bag	1	1
1	whole clove	1	1
1 pinch	cinnamon	1 pinch	1 pinch
1 pinch	nutmeg	1 pinch	1 pinch
¾ cup	boiling water	175 ml	6 fl oz
3 tbls	low-calorie cranberry juice cocktail	3 tbls	3 tbls
	sugar substitute equivalent to		
	1 tsp sugar		
1	slice of orange	1	1

Steep the tea bag and spices in the boiling water for 3 minutes. Discard the tea bag and stir in the cranberry or orange juice and sugar substitute. Add the slice of orange and serve.

* If low-calorie cranberry juice cocktail is unavailable, substitute orange juice.

Iced Tea

Serves 4 0 calories

4	tea bags	4	4
1 cup	boiling water	225 ml	8 fl oz
4	lemon wedges	4	4

Steep the tea bags in the boiling water about 5 minutes, making a strong concentration. Discard the bags and let the tea cool completely. Pour the concentrate into a large pitcher and add cold water to make up the volume to 1 qt/950 ml/1½ pt. Fill 4 tall glasses with ice cubes and pour the tea over the ice. Decorate with lemon wedges and serve, using sugar substitute to taste, if desired.

* You can, of course, make a refreshing variety of drinks by using herbal and flower teas, which are available in convenient tea-bag form. Choose from chamomile, peppermint, rose hip and many others.

Notes

MENUS

BREAKFAST (150 – 210 calories)

Omelet and salad – 170 calories

3 egg-white omelet	45
2 slices tomato	20
¼ cup/50 g/2 oz low-fat cottage cheese	50
¼ cup/50 g/2 oz chopped green pepper	15
1 thin slice wholewheat bread	40

Cereal and fruit – 175 calories

¾ cup/60 g/6 oz All-Bran, cornflakes or Rice Krispies	90
½ cup/125 ml/4 fl oz skim milk	45
1 serving fruit	40

Boiled egg and toast – 200 calories

1 soft-boiled egg	75
2 thin slices wholewheat toast	80
1 tsp margarine	45

Toast and fruit – 210 calories

French toast (with a sprinkling of artificial sweetener if liked)	170
1 serving fruit	40

Cottage cheese and fruit – 210 calories

½ cup/100 g/4 oz low-fat cottage cheese	100
1 serving fruit	40
1 thin slice wholewheat bread	40
1 tsp margarine	30

Cereal and yoghurt – 200 calories

1 serving cereal	90
¼ cup/50 g/2 oz low-fat plain yoghurt	50
1 tbls raisins	20
1 thin slice wholewheat bread	40

Porridge and toast – 185 calories

½ cup/75 g/3 oz porridge oats	70
½ cup/125 ml/4 fl oz skim milk	45
artificial sweetener, if liked	negligible
1 thin slice wholewheat bread	40
1 tsp margarine	30

NOTE: It is recommended that you add 1 tsp polyunsaturated margarine to each day's menu – spread it on bread or toast or melt it on potatoes or other vegetables. This adds 45 calories, and is thought to be helpful in lowering the blood cholesterol level

It is also advisable to take one multi-vitamin tablet each day while following this program.

FIRST WEEK

Breakfast *choose any one of the seven suggestions*

Day 1

Lunch – 260 calories

Luncheon lasagne	145
small salad and low-calorie dressing	25
1 serving fruit	40
2 tbls plain low-fat yoghurt	50

Dinner – 340 calories

Baked chicken Parmesan	230
green beans	25
Baked custard	85

Day 2

Lunch – 165 calories

Chili con carne	100
small salad and low-calorie dressing	25
1 serving fruit	40

Dinner – 385 calories

Foil-baked fish	235
½ baked or boiled potato	45
mock sour cream, 1 tbls	15
spinach	25
small salad and low-calorie dressing	
1 serving fruit	40

Day 3

Lunch – 175 calories

Vegetable beef soup, 2 servings	110
1 small salad and low-calorie dressing	25
1 serving fruit	40

Dinner – 409 calories

Madelain's company veal	294
½ baked or boiled potato	45
4 Herbed carrots	30
Baked apple	40

Day 4

Lunch – 220 calories

Spanish omelet	180
1 serving fruit	40

Dinner – 410 calories

Stuffed pepper	300
small salad and low-calorie dressing	25
½ baked or boiled potato	45
1 serving fruit	40

Day 5

Lunch – 190 calories

Macaroni and cheese casserole	125
small salad and low-calorie dressing	25
1 serving fruit	40

Dinner – 400 calories

Broccoli rice and chicken liver	360
1 serving fruit	40

Day 6

Lunch – 205 calories

50 g/2 oz shrimp or crab	70
4 tbls/50 g/2 oz catsup	30
small salad and low-calorie dressing	25
1 serving fruit	40
1 thin slice wholewheat bread	40

Dinner – 390 calories

roast beef	
100 g/4 oz cooked weight	240
½ baked or boiled potato	45
Beet and onion salad	25
Zucchini pomodoro	40
Tropical delight	40

Day 7

Lunch – 200 calories

Curried mushrooms	120
1 thin slice wholewheat toast	40
1 serving fruit	40

Dinner – 415 calories

Spanish chicken	325
broccoli	25
small salad and low-calorie dressing	25
1 serving fruit	40

SECOND WEEK

Breakfast *choose any one of the seven suggestions*

Day 1

Lunch – 185 calories

stuffed tomato	145
1 serving fruit	40

Dinner – 400 calories

Dinner in a tater	360
1 serving fruit	40

Day 2

Lunch – 165 calories

Tomato egg bake	100
small salad and low-calorie dressing	25
1 thin slice wholewheat bread	40

Dinner – 435 calories

Spaghetti with meat sauce	335
small salad and low-calorie dressing	25
Parmesan cheese, 1 tbls	35
1 serving fruit	40

Day 3

Lunch – 175 calories

Confetti cottage cheese salad	95
2 thin slices melba toast	30
lettuce	10
1 serving fruit	40

Dinner – 445 calories

Beef stroganoff with rice or noodles	380
small salad and low-calorie dressing	25
1 serving fruit	40

Day 4

Lunch – 170 calories

Cream of consommé	75
2 slices melba toast	30
small salad and low-calorie dressing	25
1 serving fruit	40

Dinner – 460 calories

Shrimp Louisianne with rice	350
Bean salad	25
Baked custard	85

Day 5

Lunch – 175 calories

Stuffed mushrooms	110
small salad and low-calorie dressing	25
thin slice wholewheat bread	40

Dinner – 440 calories

Enchilada casserole	315
Marinated vegetable salad	25
Peach custard pie	100

Day 6

Lunch – 185 calories

Stuffed baked potato	90
Beet and onion salad	25
1 serving fruit	40
2 slices melba toast	30

Dinner – 385 calories

Sautéed chicken breasts	275
spinach	25
½ baked or boiled potato	45
Frosty banana	40

Day 7

Lunch – 165 calories

Broccoli soufflé	95
2 slices melba toast	30
1 serving fruit	40

Dinner – 435 calories

broiled steak – 225 g/8 oz cooked	300
½ baked or boiled potato	45
green beans	25
Hot pineapple and yoghurt	65

THIRD WEEK

Breakfast choose any of the seven suggestions

Day 1

Lunch – 195 calories

Spinach soup	40
3 egg-white omelet	115
1 serving fruit	40

Dinner – 415 calories

Chicken curry casserole	350
cauliflower	25
1 serving fruit	40

Day 2

Lunch – 180 calories

Artichokes with herb sauce	95
2 slices melba toast	30
25 g/1 oz tuna and 1 tbls yoghurt	55

Dinner – 434 calories

Bebe's shrimp and peppers	162
½ cup/100 g/4 oz boiled rice	100
Baked spinach	132
1 serving fruit	40

Day 3

Lunch - 200 calories

Ratatouille	160
1 serving fruit	40

Dinner – 410 calories

Beef loaf	220
Cabbage in the oven	165
small salad and low-calorie dressing	25

Day 4

Lunch – 175 calories

Stuffed mushrooms	110
small salad and low-calorie dressing	25
1 serving fruit	40

Dinner – 397 calories

Foil-baked fish	235
Tomatoes in the oven	117
1 serving fruit	45

Day 5

Lunch – 195 calories

Chili con carne	100
Beet and onion salad	25
2 slices melba toast	30
1 serving fruit	40

Dinner – 390 calories

Stuffed cabbage leaves	205
½ baked or boiled potato	45
small salad and low-calorie dressing	25
Prune and orange cake	115

Day 6

Lunch – 205 calories

Spanish omelet	180
small salad and low-calorie dressing	25

Dinner – 404 calories

Paprika shrimp	229
½ cup/100 g/4 oz rice	100
green peas	35
Tropical delight	

Day 7

Lunch – 220 calories

Stir-fry vegetables and beef	195
small salad and low-calorie dressing	25

Dinner – 430 calories

Chicken of 5 seasonings	300
Stir-fry vegetables	45
½ baked or boiled potato	45
1 serving fruit	40

FOURTH WEEK

Breakfast choose any one of the seven suggestions

Day 1

Lunch – 180 calories

Stuffed baked potato	90
small salad and low-calorie dressing	25
1 serving fruit and 1 tbls plain low-fat yoghurt	65

Dinner – 435 calories

Swedish meatballs Stroganoff	310
Herbed carrots	
green beans	25
3 slices tomato	30
1 serving fruit	40

Day 2

Lunch – 200 calories

Tomato egg bake	100
small salad and low-calorie dressing	25
2 slices melba toast	30
1 serving fruit	40

Dinner – 395 calories

Scallops Hawaiian with rice	300
asparagus	25
small salad and low-calorie dressing	25
Cinnamon apple cream	45

Day 3

Lunch – 185 calories

roast beef – sliced, 50 g/2 oz cooked weight	120
1 thin slice wholewheat bread	40
mustard and lettuce	negligible
Quick vegetable soup	25

Dinner – 435 calories

Chicken oriental and rice	370
small salad and low-calorie dressing	25
1 serving fruit	40

Day 4

Lunch – 210 calories

Zucchini casserole	185
small salad and low-calorie dressing	25

Dinner – 405 calories

Company tuna casserole	230
½ baked or boiled potato	45
1 tbls plain low-fat yoghurt	20
broccoli	25
1 tbls margarine	45
1 serving fruit	40

Day 5

Lunch – 200 calories

Apple, celery and raisin salad	160
1 thin slice wholewheat bread	40

Dinner – 405 calories

Spaghetti casserole	380
small salad and low-calorie dressing	25

Day 6

Lunch – 220 calories

Tuna sandwich	180
lettuce	negligible
1 serving fruit	40

Dinner – 410 calories

Curried chicken and rice	300
green beans	25
Strawberry banana chantilly	85

Day 7

Lunch – 175 calories

Chicken salad	105
2 lettuce leaves	negligible
2 slices melba toast	30
1 serving fruit	40

Dinner – 400 calories

Three-cheese quiche	260
broccoli	
Herbed carrots	30
small salad and low-calorie dressing	25
Orange freeze	60

Index